LIFE IS HARD
FOOD IS EASY

LIFE IS HARD
FOOD IS EASY

The 5-Step Plan
to Overcome Emotional Eating
and Lose Weight on Any Diet

Linda Spangle, R.N., M.A.

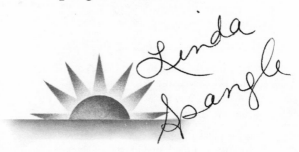

LifeLine
Press

A Regnery Publishing Company • Washington, D.C.

Library of Congress Cataloging-in-Publication Data

Spangle, Linda.
  Life is hard, food is easy : the 5-step plan to overcome emotional eating and lose weight on any diet / Linda Spangle.
    p. cm.   9/04
  Includes index.
  ISBN 0-89526-145-6 (alk. paper)
  1. Weight loss--Psychological aspects. 2. Compulsive eating. I. Title.
  RM222.2 .S636 2002   2003
  613.2'5'019--dc21

                                        2002152939

Published in the United States by
LifeLine Press
A Regnery Publishing Company
One Massachusetts Avenue, N.W.
Washington, DC 20001

Visit us at www.lifelinepress.com

Distributed to the trade by
National Book Network
4720-A Boston Way
Lanham, MD 20706

Printed on acid-free paper
Manufactured in the United States of America

10 9 8 7 6 5 4 3 2 1

Books are available in quantity for promotional or premium use. Write to Director of Special Sales, Regnery Publishing, Inc., One Massachusetts Avenue, N.W., Washington, DC 20001, for information on discounts and terms or call (202) 216-0600.

The information contained in this book is not a substitute for medical counseling and care. All matters pertaining to your physical health should be supervised by a health care professional.

To my loving husband, Mike Spangle, for always seeing
my potential instead of my struggles.

Contents

Part Three: Building Your Skills

Foreword

IN THE FIELD OF WEIGHT MANAGEMENT, one of the biggest struggles is keeping people dedicated not only to losing weight, but also to changing their lifestyle and behaviors to make a lasting difference. This book identifies many of the reasons why people struggle to make their diet plans work. Linda Spangle helps you appreciate that perhaps it's not the diet that failed you; maybe it's you that failed the diet.

As the president and CEO of Medifast, Inc., I have seen firsthand the difference Linda has made in people's lives. Since the early nineties, the Medifast weight-loss program has been used by more than 700,000 people and recommended by more than 15,000 medical practitioners. During her many years of working with Medifast, Linda Spangle has been one of the most successful clinicians in our network, mostly due to her emphasis on the emotional aspects of eating and dieting.

In her clinic, Linda developed and taught a dynamic model for behavior modification that increased her success rates dramatically. Linda's methodology along with her clinical expertise in the areas of weight management, behavior change, and emotional eating has given many of her patients new hope for long-term success.

Life Is Hard, Food Is Easy will help you understand the psychological reasons for emotional eating and teach you how to conquer old habits that get in the way of your progress. As you become more aware of how life issues affect the way you feel and even what you eat, you'll be able to learn how to overcome these challenges and build a plan that brings lasting success.

Bradley T. MacDonald
Chief Executive Officer
Medifast, Inc.

Acknowledgments

ALONG THE JOURNEY OF WRITING THIS BOOK, I've been blessed to have the support and guidance of so many people. Thanks to my publishing team at LifeLine Press, especially Mike Ward, for believing in this project and also for helping create the book title. Special thanks to my editor and friend, Molly Mullen, for your solid work as well as your ongoing encouragement.

Thanks to my feedback team, especially family therapist Lavonne Johnson, who provided valuable insight and information on the psychological issues. I'd also like to thank my friend and editor, Barbara McNichol, who always took my "perfect" work and made it so much better.

Special thanks to Medifast Inc. CEO, Colonel Brad McDonald, a true pioneer in the field of obesity treatment. For many years, your support of my WINNERS clinic and my research with overweight individuals has given my work depth and helped me serve this population better. Thanks to the entire staff at Medifast for your kindness and support, and to the medical director, Dr. Wayne Andersen, for your passion to help people become healthier.

I'd like to thank my mentor and friend, Jack Canfield, and the Self-Esteem Seminar training group. You helped me dig deeper than I knew was possible, giving me valuable skills for coaching others in their personal growth.

I wish to thank all the clients who taught me about the pain, the learning, and the joy of weight-loss success. Special thanks to Mary Jane Medlock, my coaching client who lost well over 100 pounds and has successfully maintained her weight. Thanks for openly sharing your stories and your heart as we learned together. I greatly appreciate all of the people whose experiences contributed to this book and the ways each of you helped me become a stronger support for individuals who struggle with emotional eating.

Finally, I'd like to thank my husband, Mike Spangle, for constantly reminding me that I'm a great writer, even during times when I don't believe it myself. You are always there for me, encouraging me on the good days and helping me cry on the bad ones. Your consistent love and support have been critical to my success with this book as well as my writing and teaching career. I also thank God for giving me the gift of writing and for teaching me how to help others heal the pain in their lives.

Introduction

ON THE WAY HOME FROM WORK, Kathy stopped to visit her mother. She'd planned to stay only a few minutes, but then she noticed the plate of freshly baked chocolate chip cookies. They smelled wonderful! "I'll have just one," she thought. And she did. It tasted so good that soon she reached for another, then several more.

Suddenly she caught herself. "What am I doing?" she thought. "Get those away from me!" But it was too late. Once more, she had slipped off her diet and consumed her entire day's worth of calories in one sitting.

Does this sound familiar? Do you ever follow your diet plan all day, then when evening comes, eat everything in sight? Are there days when you eat a lot of food but don't know why? What makes your dieting resolve disappear so quickly around a box of doughnuts or the restaurant dessert tray?

Think about all the reasons why you might eat something. "Because I'm hungry" will probably show up on the list. But what about all the times you reach for food when you *aren't* hungry or physically needing nourishment? See if you've recently used any of these excuses:

- I just wanted something to eat.
- It looked good, so I ate it.
- Mom made it especially for me.
- I paid for that food and I want to get my money's worth.
- I was taught to clean my plate.
- I love to eat and that food was my favorite.

Most of us would admit we sometimes reach for food when hunger has nothing to do with it. If you occasionally give in to an afternoon candy bar or take a second helping of lasagna, you probably won't cause much damage. But if you're trying to lose or maintain your weight, non-hungry eating has the potential to sabotage everything you've worked for.

Using food to appease an emotional or psychological need can easily become a habit. Without realizing it, you slide into the habit of using food to fix every emotion from anger and stress to depression and boredom. Over time, your eating plan becomes ineffective, your self-esteem drops, and your weight keeps going up.

I don't believe you need a stricter diet plan to protect you from doughnuts or chocolate chip cookies. You won't conquer emotional eating by avoiding food. Instead, you need to tackle the *source* of the problem and begin to understand *why* you so easily reach for food when you aren't hungry.

For me, learning this principle didn't come easily! When I opened my wellness clinic in 1989, I assumed that the principles of healthy nutrition, regular exercise, and behavior modification would solve most people's problems with being overweight.

But even with my diligent teaching, many of my clients would repeatedly lose weight, then gain it back. I experimented with new techniques, shifting the emphasis from "dieting" to "never diet again." I advocated throwing away the scale.

For a while, I recommended the government's food pyramid (eat bread), then I switched to a high-protein plan (don't eat bread). My clients drank liquid supplements and swallowed pills. Of course, all of these methods worked for a while. But invariably many of my clients returned, frustrated with having regained weight they'd worked so hard to lose.

My personal success wasn't much better. Like many of you, I've lost over 100 pounds—by dropping the same fifteen to twenty pounds again and again. For many years, I kept trying different diet plans, typically losing weight but eventually experiencing the same frustrating re-gain.

Finally I started thinking that maybe it wasn't the *diet* that failed. I noticed that every weight-loss plan worked as long as *I worked at it*. But when I got tired or upset or depressed, I tended to slip back into my old habits of eating to feel better. Eventually, I concluded that instead of searching for another diet, I had to change the way I handled my emotions.

I began revising my long-held philosophies and attitudes about weight loss. In my clinic, I developed creative ways to help my clients nurture themselves and build their own motivation. I challenged them to figure out what they were *feeling* and to work through their negative emotions instead of using food to shove them away.

As a result of this new direction, my clinic's success rates began to improve. In my own life, my weight stabilized and my eating patterns became less chaotic. Over the years, I've continued to develop methods for helping people learn how to identify and express their emotions instead of "eating" them.

This book is not about compulsive overeating or all-night

binges. It's written for people like you and me who raid the refrigerator after a tough day and, in ten minutes, undo an entire week's worth of careful eating. But instead of merely suggesting you eat only low-fat snacks, I'll help you figure out *why* you keep standing in front of the refrigerator in the first place.

In this book, you'll learn how to revise your entire outlook on food and eating. And most of all, you'll discover the secrets to managing your emotions and your needs without reaching for food.

Initially, we will explore some of the life patterns that hooked you into food in the first place. You will probably recognize yourself in many of the stories, and you'll begin to understand how food became so important in your life. You may also realize that to stop emotional eating, you'll need to give up using food as your best friend.

Next, I'll walk you through a series of five unique steps that will help you overcome almost any food craving or non-hungry desire to eat. You can use each step individually as an immediate strategy for managing food temptation. But you'll also benefit from going through all five steps in sequence.

Each step will add depth to your understanding of the emotions or needs behind your current food struggle. With practice, you'll be able to flash through all five steps in less than a minute, giving you an instant and powerful tool for managing your emotional needs without reaching for food.

Along with each step, you'll learn a set of skills that will almost guarantee long-term success with managing your weight. I'll show you simple ways to perk up your self-esteem, manage people who make you crazy, and tackle those areas where you set yourself up for failure. As you integrate the materials from this book into your life, you'll realize how simple it is to make any diet or weight-loss plan work.

Eventually, you'll no longer need to eat your way through a bad day or a relationship breakup. Instead, you'll discover how to identify and label the emotions that prompt your eating desires. As you become clear on what you're feeling, you'll be able to take care of what's missing in your life instead of asking food to do it for you.

By managing both food *and* your emotions, you'll be able to go through your days without feeling remorse about everything you eat. Most of all, you'll learn how to handle those times when life is hard without making food the "easy" solution.

PART ONE

TAKE POWER OVER FOOD

CHAPTER ONE

Food Is My Best Friend

LET'S GET ONE THING STRAIGHT. Food is wonderful! There's absolutely nothing wrong with food or with enjoying it. Food helps us relax, gives us ways to celebrate, and connects us with our family and friends. It fixes our bad days and brightens our good ones. Most of us love getting together with other people to share food, talk about food, and joke about how stuffed we feel after eating too much food.

If we could just separate food and eating from how we cope with life, most of us wouldn't have problems with gaining weight. But all too often, food becomes an easy solution to dealing with our uncomfortable emotions. It also replaces what's missing in our lives—things like attention, pleasure, or loving relationships.

What Is Emotional Eating?

It starts innocently enough. You open a box of Girl Scout cookies, planning to eat just a couple. An hour later, you realize you've finished off half the box. Or perhaps at a party, you reach into a bowl of peanuts or M&Ms® and quickly lose track of how many times you grab another handful.

Maybe you don't consider these eating patterns to be related to your emotions. But think about how often you put food into your mouth when you aren't physically hungry or needing a meal. Here's how I define emotional eating: *Using food for emotional or psychological reasons instead of for satisfying the body's physical requirement for food.*

Sneaking candy from the jar on your coworker's desk, appreciating the homemade cookies in the break room, or eating ice cream every night at bedtime all fit this description. The food somehow meets a need or fills a gap in your life.

Emotional eating can be obvious, like when you hunt for a snack when you feel stressed or angry. But sometimes the connection is more hidden and harder to recognize. All of the following situations qualify as emotional eating.

When the kids go down for their naps, I start searching the cupboards. I'm not hungry, I just want to eat something. —Peggy

I can't break my habit of stopping for a Big Mac and fries on the way home from work. Since I don't want my family to know, I always eat a full dinner with them as well. —John

My therapist is helping me work through some difficult issues including a history of incest and my husband's death from alcohol and drug problems. Recently, after an extremely painful counseling session, I decided to go to a movie. I kept thinking about how I wanted a large popcorn with lots of butter, a giant Coke, and a box of Raisinettes. It didn't matter which movie I would go to—I just wanted an acceptable way to justify eating all that food. —Anne

You probably recognize when you're slipping into emotional eating. But stopping the pattern of using food to fix your emotional needs may feel nearly impossible. Even if you're ready to change, you may not know how to replace what food does for you.

The Cost of Emotional Eating

There's no question that food does make us feel better, at least temporarily. But real life is still there when we stop eating. At some point, the pleasure ends and negative feelings creep in. Guilt and remorse don't stop us; they just lead to more eating. As a weight-loss counselor, I've watched many people struggle to change this pattern.

In her journal, Paula described how food helps her avoid the harsh realities of her situation.

Life didn't turn out the way I planned. I thought I'd meet a gorgeous guy, have an exciting career, two or three brilliant children, and a beautiful house. Instead, here I am, twice divorced, stuck living in this dumpy basement apartment. I feel trapped in my job because I can't afford to go back to school.

When I'm alone at night, feeling angry at life and disgusted with my fat self, eating helps me forget all of this. I desperately wish it was different. But when I sit on my faded couch with my friends Ben and Jerry, I can briefly ignore how my life sucks.

Tonight, I'm digging into a pint of New York Super Fudge Chunk. I mash those chocolate pieces with my teeth, lick the fudge off my lips, and slide into feeling comforted. Of course, my weight keeps going up and my life never improves, but I'll do this again tomorrow night. I hate living this way, but I have no idea how to stop. —Paula

Perhaps your story isn't as extreme as Paula's. But you probably recognize the pattern of using food to fix many of the negative things in your life. Sandy has tried many diet plans over the years. But her success never lasts because she always slips back into a predictable cycle of eating, feeling bad, then eating again. Here's how she describes her pattern:

First I eat to calm down and relax at the end of a hard day. As the evening drags on, I eat because I'm alone and bored. Later, I eat because I'm frustrated and disgusted with myself. Once again, I've completely blown my diet and I feel awful. So then I eat to punish myself for being bad and for screwing up my goals. I tell myself, "It's your own fault you are so fat. You don't deserve to be thin, so shove this pastry down your throat." —Sandy

How Food Became Hooked to Emotions

We didn't start out being emotional eaters. As babies, we cried for food when we were hungry, and when we'd had enough, we drifted off to sleep. But somehow, in the process of growing up, this simple way of life began to shift. Food started showing up everywhere, and it didn't seem to matter whether we were hungry or not, we ate anyway.

One of my favorite childhood memories comes from our Sunday noon meals at home. I grew up on a working farm and on Sundays we often had visitors. The table was usually loaded with platters of fried chicken along with bowls of gravy, mashed potatoes, and fresh, sweet corn. We always finished with homemade apple pie or a three-layer chocolate cake.

I loved those Sundays. I can't remember exact details of how the food tasted, but I know we had fun. Mom smiled a lot as she watched us stuff ourselves with her cooking. As I pushed back from the table afterward, I would feel so good—too full, of course, but satisfied, warm, and loved.

Food meant happiness at our house. Around the dinner table, we would tell jokes and silly stories that made our mother laugh until tears ran down her cheeks. At family gatherings, food helped us celebrate everything—birthdays, holidays, even just the end of a long week.

You may have grown up with similar food connections. As a child, you probably didn't associate food with emotions or problems. Mostly, you just ate your meals and ran out to play, giving little thought to what you had eaten.

Then things began to change. On your birthday, you blew out the candles and everyone celebrated by eating chocolate cake. People encouraged you, "Eat more, it's good for you," and they applauded you for cleaning your plate.

If you fell down, Mom gave you a cookie and your skinned knee magically stopped hurting. After baseball and soccer, you ate pizza whether you won the game or lost. Food added pleasure to either outcome. You learned that food could turn anything into a fun event or fix any experience that didn't come out quite right.

In contrast, food may also have served as a method of control, rewarding when you were good and punishing if you weren't. Maybe you heard, "If you pick up your toys, I'll give you a snack" or "No dessert until you clean your plate." Perhaps you recall being sent to bed with no dinner because you had "misbehaved."

If you were overweight as a child, you may have endured restrictions to your food and eating patterns. You may still cringe at the words, "You can't have that! It will make you fat." Extreme rules about eating may have taught you to sneak food or find other ways to get the treats you wanted.

The Comfort of Food

Many people discovered very early that food could protect them from painful situations or help them feel safe. Maybe you crawled into bed and nibbled from a bag of potato chips while you read steamy romance novels. In the safety of your room, the food made it easier to ignore the fighting or yelling that went on in your home.

It doesn't take a traumatic event or a bad childhood to get hooked into eating for emotional reasons. But at some point, you probably faced a difficult situation and thought, "If I eat something, maybe I'll feel better." And you did.

Over the years, repeating this experience created a link between food and your emotions. But once you become hooked into emotional eating, you can lose sight of how much it affects you.

FOOD AS CONSOLATION PRIZE

You keep hoping that one of these days food will provide what you really need in life. But it doesn't. Eventually, overeating numbs your emotions and you stop noticing what's missing. Food provides a legal, socially acceptable way to escape from reality.

But even though eating may temporarily soothe an emotional need, the end result never matches your dream. Food becomes the *consolation prize*—better than nothing, but not even close to what you really wanted, which was to be loved, appreciated, comforted, or encouraged.

Many days, we'd give anything for someone to hold us or to offer kind, encouraging words. We want somebody to care that we have a bad cold or that our car broke down for the third time this month. We wish our lives were different—that we had more money, more love, or more fun. When we don't get these things, it's easy to look for something to take the place of what's missing.

On Friday night, I planned to go to a movie, but when I got to the theater, the show was sold out. So I stopped at the video store on the way home and rented a movie instead. It turned out to be horrible—not the slightest bit entertaining or enjoyable. But the evening wasn't a total loss. I had my pint of Häagen-Dazs, so that became my fun. —Don

Whenever we go through major changes in life, food provides an anchor. As we scramble to adjust to new surroundings, we realize that food doesn't change. We can travel anywhere, go to any job, move to a new apartment, and food is still there! It makes us feel secure because it's something familiar.

FOOD AS SURVIVAL

Many overweight people admit they use food as a drug, hoping to escape their uncomfortable thoughts and feelings. In her job as a human resources director, Alice became skilled at resolving personnel conflicts and creating solutions to work problems. All day long she takes care of other people and addresses their concerns. But she admits that once she gets home, food is her solace, giving her the comfort and validation that are missing in her work life. Alice told me, "I don't eat food; I use food! But I don't know how to survive without it."

Peter fears that if he couldn't use food for comfort, he wouldn't be able to cope.

For me, overeating is like pushing the "mute" button on my life. But I keep doing it, because if I stop, life feels too awful to deal with. —Peter

Food Was My Best Friend

In my own life, it took me many years to learn that eating to feel better doesn't change anything. For a long time, I managed painful emotions by stuffing them deep inside with food. But before I could change this pattern, I had to recognize and acknowledge what I was doing. My journey began after nine years of silence, a time in which I never spoke of my personal pain and instead used food to push my feelings far away.

Despite years of intense efforts, my husband and I do not have children. I was born with an abnormally shaped uterus that cannot support a full-term pregnancy. Doctors tried everything possible to help me bear children. I went through several major surgeries, spent months in bed, and endured painful hormone shots.

Three different times, I carried a pregnancy for six months before going into premature labor. Two of my baby girls were stillborn. The third one lived for eleven hours before her tiny lungs quit working. Complications with the final pregnancy prevented me from ever being able to try again.

When I learned I would never be able to have children, I was devastated. My sadness lingered for years and, in fact, it has never faded completely. For a time, my husband and I considered adopting, but finances and a variety of other factors kept this from happening. So we made the decision to accept we wouldn't have children and to move on with our lives.

To cope with my grief, I stayed very busy, immersing myself in my work as a nurse and health educator. For the next nine years, I rarely spoke about my loss or told people what I'd been through. Discussing the loss of the babies made me cry, so I just didn't allow myself to talk about it.

Whenever I felt sad about my babies, I would eat a lot and try to avoid thinking. Because soft foods felt especially comforting, I ate lots of doughnuts and noodle casseroles. My weight-loss efforts never lasted because I spent so much time eating away the painful memories of losing my babies.

MOTHER'S DAY EATING

Mother's Day has always been a difficult holiday for me. On this day, when my friends are enjoying homemade cards and breakfast in bed, my disappointment and grief return with a vengeance. For many years, I would eat all day long on Mother's Day, trying to pretend the holiday didn't exist.

One year, after I'd battled an extensive winter depression, a counselor suggested I stop avoiding the emotions of Mother's Day and instead allow myself to feel them. I was terrified by the thought, but I decided to follow her advice. With my counselor's help, I planned that I would let my grief surface, then acknowledge it instead of eating to push it away.

That Mother's Day morning, I woke up determined I would not use food to stop my feelings. I drank coffee and ate a small breakfast. Then I waited. Late in the morning, I felt the sadness rising—the deep painful emotions I'd always tried to avoid. But this time, I let them come. When the tears started, I sat at my kitchen table, buried my head in my arms, and sobbed for an hour.

I cried for everything I missed by not having my babies. I wept for not taking them to their first day of kindergarten or picking out prom dresses or watching them cross the stage at graduations. I grieved for never getting to plan their weddings and I mourned that I would never have grandchildren. I shed tears for all the love and the memories that never got a chance to exist. I hurt for the sadness I saw in my husband. I cried for myself, and for the ache that had never left the deepest corner of my heart.

Finally, I was quiet. Shakily I got up from the table, washed my face, and went outside into the sunshine. As I stood in the warmth, I felt an amazing sense of calm. And I realized I had no desire to eat. Expressing those sad emotions had let me feel the pain and survive it without needing to rely on casseroles or brownies.

That day, I turned a corner in my life. From then on, I started *encouraging* my emotions instead of stopping them. Little by little, I learned to allow other painful feelings to surface and to express them in ways that moved me toward healing.

Much of what you will read in this book comes from my ongoing personal growth. Emotional eating never completely loses its power and it still seduces me as a way to make life easier. When times are difficult or I'm feeling down, I occasionally slip into nurturing myself with cookies or a doughnut. But I keep striving to recognize my feelings and manage them *before* I reach my hand out for food.

From Harmful to Healthy

When food routinely fills the emptiness in your life, it slips into the role of being your best friend. You can always count on food to be there for you and to take care of you. But at the same time you're comforting yourself with cheesecake or potato chips, you secretly know this friendship is ruining your life.

It's time for a change. In this book, you will learn how to analyze what you need and how to label your emotions accurately. You'll have a chance to practice expressing your feelings and coping with them in ways that don't involve using food. As you become aware of what you truly need in life and develop skills to fill those needs, you'll be able to change your friendship with food into a healthy relationship.

I still cry on Mother's Day. But instead of running from my sadness with a bag of doughnuts in my hand, I wait for the tears and embrace them when they come. I allow myself to cry as long as I need to, and when I'm done, I remind myself that I've taken another step in my emotional healing.

You can find this strength, too. Start by realizing that the key to managing your weight begins with healing your heart, not filling your spoon. As you discover new ways to cope with the emotional issues of life, you'll move toward a sense of peace with food—a feeling you may have forgotten existed.

Food is wonderful!
In fact, food is my best friend,
but lately I'm aware that
my friend is hurting me,
making me uncomfortable,
sabotaging my goals,
causing me grief and guilt,
possibly destroying my life.
Today I made a decision—
it's time to get a new friend.

—Linda Spangle

CHAPTER TWO

Put Food in Its Place

BEFORE YOU BEGIN WORKING on your emotional coping patterns, let's review a few basic principles about managing food. And here's the good news—you don't have to give up the pleasure of eating in order to manage your weight. By making a few simple changes in how you approach food, you can learn how to eat *anything* without damaging your diet plan.

The "New" Purpose of Food

Think about all the situations when your food intake has nothing to do with hunger or nutritional needs. As you move toward managing emotional eating, you may need to redefine how you approach food, including *why* and *when* you will eat. In other words, you need to put food in its place!

From now on, determine that you'll eat for only two purposes: to fuel your body and to appreciate flavors. Measure all of your intake against these two guidelines. If your reason for putting something in your mouth doesn't match either one, you are probably doing emotional eating.

Fuel Your Body

Just like your car, your body needs fuel to keep it moving efficiently. To get the best mileage out of your body, you'll want to fill your tank at intervals, stop when it's full, and use high-quality fuel. If you ignore "empty tank" signals like hunger or other physical signs of needing fuel, you're more likely to overeat or give in to food temptations.

DON'T SKIP MEALS

Give your body something to run on! Plan to get a minimum of three fuel stops a day, with optional mini-stops in between. You don't need to eat a lot at each fueling. In fact, many people do well by eating five or six times a day, dividing their food into small meals and healthy snacks.

Be sure to keep your fuel intake consistent. Not eating breakfast, eating at odd times, or going too long between meals can contribute to weight *gain* rather than weight loss. Your body views long periods of not eating as similar to a famine, so it protects itself by storing calories for later use.

When she's planning to go out for a big dinner at night, Susan avoids eating all day. She says she's "saving up" the calories so she'll have lots of room for her favorite foods. Unfortunately, this pattern may do the opposite of what Susan intended. Even though she eats about the same number of calories as usual, her body may store part of what she eats in the evening, causing her to gain weight.

DON'T GET TOO HUNGRY

If you let your tank go too long, you may lose your resolve to eat right. The hungrier you get, the greater the risk you'll eat too much, make poor food choices, and—worst of all—not care! Dur-

ing your waking hours, use a "five-hour rule" to help monitor your
fuel level. If you go longer than five hours without food, you'll
increase your chances of overeating when you finally do eat.

Hunger or a "desire to eat"? When food thoughts pop into
your mind, determine whether they are related to true physical
hunger or to a "desire to eat." Real hunger generally shows up as a
growling, hollow feeling in your stomach or maybe a slight headache.
But if you start pacing around the kitchen an hour after you finish
lunch, you're probably dealing with a desire to eat, not actual hunger.

Don't convince yourself you need food when you're just restless or trying to avoid a task. Label your search for what it is—in
this case, wanting to eat instead of doing your work.

How morning affects evening. Do you ever start munching
late in the day, then snack your way through the rest of the afternoon and evening? If you struggle with late-day hunger, fatigue, or
food cravings, the culprit may be how you ate in the morning.

When you don't get enough fuel during the early part of the
day, by late afternoon your body starts screaming for food. Worse
yet, your system may have a hard time catching up, making you
want to keep eating even after you've finished a large meal.

To break this pattern, space your fuel stops more frequently
during the first half of the day. Eat a mini-meal or a healthy snack
in the middle of the afternoon to prevent yourself from getting too
hungry and overeating at dinner.

FUEL OR FILLER?

Quality fuel should provide solid, lasting energy. When you exist
on low-nutrient foods such as cookies or chips, you put "filler" into
your tank, which makes it hard to get very good mileage. Don't ask
your body to run on junk. Poor-quality fuel takes a toll on your
energy as well as your weight-management efforts.

REASONABLE AMOUNTS

Do you tend to overfuel your body just a little every day? You may need to get back in touch with the size of your fuel tank and what constitutes a "reasonable amount" of food. Even if you don't know exactly how much intake your body requires, you probably recognize when you've eaten an "unreasonable" amount.

Most people need some type of measurement system to track the amounts they eat. You might count calories or fat grams or record all of your food intake. But you can also manage food volume by avoiding second helpings or limiting snacks to the amount that fits in the palm of your hand.

Half-off special. One effective way to monitor your intake is what I call the "half-off special." Simply eat half as much as you normally would or limit yourself to half of what you actually want.

When facing a pan of lasagna, picture the large serving you would usually eat, then take half that much. If you want a cookie, cut it into two pieces and eat only one of them. Divide your lunch sandwich in half, adding a piece of fruit to complete your meal. If you don't feel satisfied when you've finished, save the leftover food for at least two hours, then decide if you're still hungry.

If you can't stop yourself from eating the second half, you may need to look carefully at your emotional needs. When you continue eating after you've satisfied your fuel requirement, something else in your life probably needs attention or needs to be "filled."

Stop wasting food. Do you still hold a membership in the "Clean-Plate Club"? When you fill your car with gas, you don't keep pumping once the tank is full, spilling the fuel on the ground. So why would you do this with your body? Here's a new way to look at this problem: *Every time you eat food that your body doesn't need, you're wasting it!*

So now you have a choice. You can get rid of leftover food by throwing it away or by eating it. Either way, it doesn't escape the fate of being wasted. If you struggle with "clean your plate" messages, retrain yourself gradually by leaving one small piece of food uneaten at every meal. Stop giving food so much power that you can't leave some of it behind. Your weight and your health are more important than a leftover piece of cake.

Restaurant leftovers. At restaurants, you can always have your leftover food wrapped, then use it for a meal the next day. But look carefully at what you're taking with you when you do this. Restaurant meals are often higher in fat and calories than what you might ordinarily eat, so when you take your leftovers home, you end up eating excess calories twice instead of just once.

Here's an interesting experiment. Next time you go to a restaurant, notice whether the people using take-out boxes appear to be normal weight or overweight. You might get a new perspective on which group resists throwing food away.

Eat to Appreciate Flavors

At a local Starbucks coffee shop, I watched a tiny blond girl about three years old carefully balance a plastic box in her hands. As she made her way through the crowd, the top of the container unexpectedly popped open, revealing the fresh cinnamon roll inside. Her eyes widened as she gazed down at it. Then, in a voice tinged with awe, she exclaimed, "Yummy!" Her face reflected total joy and pleasure as she anticipated her treat.

Wouldn't it be wonderful to experience that level of enjoyment with your food? Eating to appreciate flavors is not the same as wolfing down your food, declaring how much you love to eat. It's allowing yourself to enjoy the taste, the texture, and the sensations

One Pea at a Time

Jan was raised in a family that had strict rules about never throwing food away. As an adult, she held on to this pattern, even when it meant she would overeat. One evening, she decided to leave one green pea on her dinner plate. Each of the next several nights, she left a little more food, increasing the amount each time by the size of a pea. Eventually, Jan broke her old habit of feeling anxious or guilty if she didn't clean her plate.

---

of the food without immediately punishing yourself because of the calories. When you choose to eat a food you love, approach it like the little blonde girl did, with amazement and delight.

SLOW DOWN

Do you tend to eat so fast your taste buds never get a chance to notice the food? To appreciate flavors, you have to slow your eating down. Otherwise it's like trying to notice the scenery while you're driving eighty miles an hour. You might proclaim how much you "love it," but you'll probably miss a lot of the details.

Here's an easy way to train yourself to eat more slowly. At the start of your meal, set a timer or the alarm on your watch for twenty minutes. Pace yourself (even if you're having just a sandwich) so you will be finishing the last bite of your food when the time is up. You may be surprised at how hard it is to make a meal last this long.

FLAVOR OR TEXTURE?

Are you sure you love the *flavor* of some foods or do you actually crave the *texture*? Sometimes we enjoy the "sensation of eating" more than the food itself. Have you ever noticed that some days you want the chewiness of a steak and other times you can't wait to sink your teeth into a soft doughnut or a cinnamon roll? Foods with an appealing texture give you pleasure by the way they *feel* in your mouth as you eat them.

Consider the difference between a strip of beef jerky and an ice cream cone. Compare the texture of macaroni and cheese to a piece of barbecued chicken. Mentally picture eating cashews, then switch to peanut butter. Notice how the texture of a food contributes to the enjoyment of eating it. In fact, some foods don't have much actual flavor, but the texture keeps us reaching for more.

THE MYTH OF "LOVING TO EAT"

"I just love to eat!"

How many times have you blamed this for your weight struggles? But stop for a minute and think about what you really love. Are you thrilled with the exquisite flavors and textures of the food? Or are you enjoying the way it feels as it slides down your throat?

Sometimes food becomes a substitute for the lack of power in other areas of your life. Do you get a sense of accomplishment when you finish off a huge steak or a plate of pasta? You may be enjoying the sensation of "conquering" the food. It's as though food is the enemy—and you beat it!

Most of us will certainly admit we like to eat and that we enjoy food. But there's a difference between appreciating the *flavor* of wonderful food and liking the way you *feel* as you eat it. "Loving to eat" may provide an excuse for the way food appeases emotional holes in your life.

WHEN FOOD DISAPPOINTS YOU

Someone at the office brought one of your favorites—a three-layer chocolate cake. You're sure it will taste wonderful and you salivate in anticipation. But once you start eating, you notice the cake is a little dry and it doesn't taste as good as you thought it would. Instead of stopping, you keep eating more, hoping it will somehow get better. Maybe you even reach for a second piece. After you finish eating, you feel disgusted with yourself and disappointed because the cake never did match the flavor or texture you wanted.

Any time a food doesn't taste as good as you expected, *stop eating it!* Or at least decide whether it's worth the extra calories to eat something you don't even enjoy. Then get rid of the rest immediately so you don't reach for it again to see if it's gotten any better!

If you keep eating a food after you realize you aren't enjoying the taste, you are slipping into a form of emotional eating. It's as though wanting your favorite food is "bad," so you force yourself to eat something you don't like.

THE FIRST TWO BITES

How much food does it take to be able to appreciate how something tastes? Actually, very little. You may not realize it, but the *first two bites* of any food have the most flavor. If you keep eating after that, you're just "feeding." Of course, if you are physically hungry, eating more food serves a purpose. But if you're eating to appreciate the flavor, then no matter how much you eat, the taste won't become any more wonderful than those first two bites. Not only do those first bites have the most impact on your taste buds, they're also the only ones that have any *nurturing* power! You'll get whatever you want from the food in those first two bites.

For example, if you're eating to feel nurtured or calmed, you'll experience some level of those feelings right away. But continuing to eat won't bring you additional relief. At some point, you'll probably feel disappointed or frustrated with your behavior instead of healed by the food.

Last night I was sitting on the couch eating a quart of Rocky Road ice cream straight from the carton. With each spoonful I kept thinking, "Maybe this is the bite that will do it." Of course, it never worked and I just felt worse. —Debra

CONSCIOUS EATING

Chuck had developed the habit of doing a lot of things at the same time he ate dinner. He would usually read the paper, watch the news on TV, and try to talk with his family while he was eating. Often he was so unaware of his food that he'd finish his meal without realizing it. His family always laughed when he searched frantically for the bread he'd already eaten, exclaiming, "Who ate my biscuit?"

How often do you eat without being aware of your actions? You can do a lot of damage with "unconscious eating," sometimes not even realizing that it's contributing to your weight gain. When you eat for fuel, staying conscious of what you're eating helps you recognize when your tank is full. And if your goal is to appreciate flavors, you want to be sure you notice the taste of what you are eating.

Do I Really Love This Food?

Try this exercise next time you dig into a food you would typically "love." Take a small bite of the food and ask yourself how it tastes. Is it good? Wonderful? Just fair?

Take another bite, asking the same questions. Is the temperature perfect or is it a little too warm or too cold?

Evaluate what you like best about this food. Is it the taste, the texture, the seasonings? Do you like how it feels in your mouth? Determine whether the food is meeting your expectations. Is it truly awesome or do you feel a bit disappointed with it? Next, decide if the food is enjoyable enough to continue eating. If you realize it's not tasting great, STOP! Don't keep eating, hoping it will get better—because it won't.

To build awareness of your actions around food, take a close look at where and when you eat. Do you use the drive-through window at a fast-food restaurant, then devour your sandwich while you're on the road? While it might feel like you are saving time, it's easy to eat without realizing you're doing it.

The disappearing candy bar. Dave was driving to a business appointment when he began thinking about a candy bar. Something chocolate and chewy sounded good. He noticed his car was low on gas, so he stopped at a convenience store to fill the tank. When he paid for the gas, he also bought two Snickers candy bars.

Back on the road, Dave listened to the radio and contemplated his strategy for the upcoming meeting. Suddenly he glanced down at the passenger seat and noticed an empty wrapper. "Wait a minute...," he thought. "I don't remember eating that candy bar!" Since there was no one else in the car, he knew *he* must have eaten it, but he had no recollection of either the flavor or the texture of the candy. Worse yet, he still wanted a Snickers, so he ate the second bar, too.

By eating unconsciously, Dave didn't get much enjoyment or satisfaction from the candy bar, leaving him still yearning for the taste. It's much easier to appreciate the flavors, textures, and sensations of a food when you pay attention to it. You are also more likely to feel satisfied, which helps you avoid eating more.

Improving your awareness. Many weight-loss books suggest you avoid doing other activities like reading or watching TV while you are eating. I'm not sure this is necessary. These days, most of us tend to multi-task by working on the computer, talking on the phone, and cleaning the house all at the same time.

Staying aware of your food doesn't *require* that you do nothing else when you eat. Instead, you simply need to remind yourself that you're eating, then notice the bites you're putting into your mouth.

Make an effort to stay focused on your food, even if you watch TV or do other activities while you are eating.

Eating with awareness gives you an amazing amount of enjoyment and satisfaction. And when you get what you wanted from the food, your craving usually stops and you discover you don't need to keep eating more.

Next time you eat a favorite food, savor it carefully. Take small bites, about the size of a fourth of a teaspoon, and pay careful attention to the food as you eat it. Notice if it's matching the taste you expected and evaluate whether you want to keep eating. Savoring works especially well with sweet things and desserts, but it can also give you a fresh appreciation for foods like green beans, cheeses, or pasta.

SMALLER AMOUNTS, LESS OFTEN

You don't need to eliminate *all* the foods you love in order to manage your weight. Make a list of your favorite high-calorie or high-fat foods, then consider including them in your diet with the following guideline: *smaller amounts, less often.* Decide ahead of time what constitutes a "smaller amount," as well as how often you will eat the food.

Suppose you normally eat a large bowl of ice cream every night. To follow your new guideline, you might plan to have ice cream just once a week and to limit the amount to one-half cup or a small cone. All week, you can look forward to your treat, and because you know you can have it eventually, you won't be as likely to feel deprived.

Sandra used this principle to manage one of her favorite foods, barbecued ribs.

There's a great restaurant close to my home that serves wonderful barbecued ribs. Right before I'd start any new diet, I would go eat a pound of those ribs because I knew I wouldn't get to have them again for months. Of course, once I fell off my diet plan, I'd reward myself with eating them again.

Using the "smaller amounts, less often" principle, I decided to fit the barbecued ribs into my eating plan once each month, and to limit my serving size to a quarter-pound. The first month I could hardly wait. I thought a lot about the ribs and how good they would taste. But since I knew they were coming, I waited for the end of the month.

When the day finally arrived, I went to the restaurant, ate the ribs, and really loved my dinner. They tasted great, and because I knew I could have them again soon, I was able to stop at my designated serving amount.

The next month, I anxiously waited for my special night out when I could eat my favorite ribs again. But this time I noticed they didn't taste quite as good as before. By the end of the third month, I didn't seem to crave them as much and I decided to go out for chicken instead. —Sandra

Savoring

Here's a simple technique to help you eat with more awareness and be sure you get what you want from your food. My favorite candy for this exercise is a little three-layer Andes-brand mint. Unwrap the mint and begin eating it slowly, biting off each of the corners, one at a time. As you eat, notice how the candy feels in your mouth. Pay special attention to the separate flavors of chocolate and mint as well as the texture.

Next, eat half of what's left, then finish the mint. You should get a total of six bites from the candy. As you finish, focus on the sensation of swallowing. Picture the mint sliding down your throat and into your stomach. Let yourself "feel" the candy as well as taste it. Once you finish this exercise, ask yourself if you want another mint. Usually, the answer is "no."

By telling herself she would always get to have those barbecued ribs, Sandra took away their power. Over time, they didn't tempt her as much and she was able to manage them better.

When you give yourself permission to eat something, you put yourself in charge of the food instead of letting it control you. Using the guidelines of "smaller amounts, less often," plan your favorite foods into your diet program. By knowing you can have them again, you will be able to wait for the designated time and then eat them in reasonable amounts.

———

As you begin your work on conquering emotional eating, use the guidelines in this chapter to help manage your daily eating plan. By using the skills of eating only to fuel your body or to appreciate flavors, you can enjoy the foods you love without gaining weight.

PART TWO

The 5-Step Plan to Overcome Emotional Eating

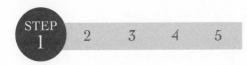

CHAPTER THREE

What's Going On?

IT'S THE MIDDLE OF THE AFTERNOON and you still haven't finished the report that's due at five o'clock. Suddenly you feel like eating something—one of those nut-filled candy bars from the vending machine sounds great. You trudge down the hall, get the candy bar, and eat half of it before you return to your desk.

Later that evening you flip through the channels on TV, but nothing looks interesting. You're exhausted from work and you wish you weren't living alone. You wander around the house thinking about eating something, but you can't decide what you want. You peek into the refrigerator to see if anything looks good. Finally you pull out the half-empty carton of caramel fudge ice cream and take a few bites. It tastes nice—kind of soothing. So you take the carton with you as you stroll back to the couch.

These eating situations involve two different types of emotional needs. The first is related to the pressures of stress and time, while the second is prompted by fatigue and boredom. In both cases, the food you selected gives clues to the emotional needs behind your eating.

In my weight-management work, I've discovered that food choices often act as a mirror, showing exactly which emotions are prompting our desire to eat. *Not knowing* what we want also points toward specific emotional needs. In this first step of conquering emotional eating, you will learn how to assess what's causing you to look for food.

Knowing what's prompting your eating desire gives you a much greater chance of doing something that will address your real need and keep you out of the cupboard. Or, if you've already eaten something, you can *look backward* and figure out what contributed to your eating and how you could prevent that situation in the future.

Whenever you recognize a non-hungry desire to eat, STOP and ask yourself what's affecting you at that moment. By analyzing your immediate situation, you can jump to an alternate plan of action and *avoid* eating.

Head Hunger or Heart Hunger?

Some years ago, I worked in a challenging job as a hospital health educator. During that time, nearly every afternoon I would get an intense craving for a cookie. So on my break, I'd walk to a nearby bakery and buy a couple of chewy oatmeal raisin cookies. It bothered me that I couldn't break this habit. But no matter how hard I tried to resist, those cookies would occupy my thoughts until I got out to the bakery for my "fix."

One afternoon, when work had been particularly stressful, I noticed I was practically gnashing my teeth as I bit into the chewy cookie. Suddenly it hit me that what I *really* wanted to chew on was my obnoxious boss and the hospital's administrative staff.

After that, I began paying attention to how I felt when I ate certain foods and I discovered some interesting connections. I noticed that when I felt stressed or frustrated, I looked for "chewy" foods like cookies or candy bars. But when I was struggling with sadness or grief, I preferred soft ones like ice cream or my own homemade macaroni casseroles.

When I explored this theory with my clients, I discovered these food categories consistently matched their experiences too. For example, when fighting stress, anger, or frustration, people typically reached for foods that were chewy or crunchy. They really wanted to "chew" on something in life—their employers, their children, or even projects or deadlines. Because this pressure-related eating seemed to be generated by specific thoughts or attitudes, I labeled it *head hunger*.

Other times, my clients would describe eating to cope with hollow or restless feelings like boredom, depression, or loneliness. When experiencing these "empty" emotions, they typically chose soft, creamy-textured foods or "comfort foods" like ice cream, pasta, or chocolate. Because this type of eating seemed connected to the "lack" of things, such as love or attention, I labeled it *heart hunger*.

With practice, you can learn how to distinguish easily between these two types of emotional eating. Once you identify what's driving your desire to eat, you can take care of what you *really* need, instead of burying your emotions under a plate of brownies or in a bag of potato chips.

These food–emotion connections may not always work for you. Sometimes you won't be able to identify any emotional issues that appear related to your eating. But keep searching. Eventually, the connection between food and your emotions will become more obvious.

Head Hunger

Head hunger usually begins with a *specific* food thought or craving. You know *exactly* what you want—a candy bar, potato chips, or perhaps that granola-nut mix left over from your camping trip. Your craving may be so precise that you make a special trip to the grocery store for your favorite brand of macadamia-nut cookies. With head hunger, some people will do whatever it takes to satisfy a food thought, even getting up in the middle of the night and driving to a fast-food restaurant.

CHEWY OR CRUNCHY FOODS

When you experience head hunger, you typically look for foods that are *chewy* or *crunchy*. Snack foods like potato chips, nuts, and candy work great. The crunchiness of these foods and the effort required to chew them provide "mouth satisfaction."

Foods with a dense, chewy texture also work for appeasing head hunger. Hamburgers, pizza, and chocolate all have a "smash-in-your-mouth" sensation that replaces what you'd really like to do to somebody or something else. From the list below, identify which foods you are most likely to reach for when you experience a sudden craving.

With head hunger, cravings often pop up quickly. One minute you feel fine, the next minute you desperately want a bag of

Common Head-Hunger Foods

Chewy Foods	Crunchy Foods	Texture Foods
Candy bars, M&Ms®	Nuts	French fries
Steak, chewy meat	Breakfast cereal	Hot dogs
Trail mix, granola	Popcorn	Pizza
Fried foods	Crackers	Chocolate

peanuts or a candy bar. When you eat in response to head hunger, you usually know when you're done. After you wolf down a cheeseburger or finish off a bag of chips, you feel better for the moment. The food soothes your intense emotions and temporarily leaves you feeling calmer or more peaceful.

WHAT DO I WANT TO "CHEW ON"?

When you recognize that you want a chewy or crunchy food, take a quick inventory of what might be bothering you. Ask yourself, "What do I really want to chew on? What's irritating, stressing, or frustrating me right now?" Your answer might include kids, finances, friends, project deadlines, or a difficult job.

I assumed it was habit sending me down the hall to the candy machine every day. Then I realized that, by the middle of the afternoon, I'd used up my patience with this job and my overbearing boss. I would eat a candy bar or two just to get through the last few hours of my day. —Marty

Pressure emotions. Head hunger is usually prompted by pressure-type emotions like anger, frustration, or resentment. Stress, deadlines, and people tend to be some of the most common reasons for head-hunger eating. When your tension level builds, you look for a quick way to get relief.

Stress and pressure make you feel impatient. Like an ice-cold drink on a blazing hot day, you want something that will take effect now. You've probably learned techniques to help you manage stress, but sometimes they seem like too much work. You don't want to take time to play relaxing music, do yoga, or take a walk. Food is easier, a lot faster, and certainly much more fun!

Whenever you reach for food to help you "calm down," recognize that head hunger is driving your behavior. Even a series of small irritations can lead to head-hunger eating. The car won't start, the supply shipment didn't arrive, you got mud on your new coat, and your four-year-old has a runny nose so she can't go to daycare. Hassles stack on top of each other like building blocks until eventually the pile topples over. When you "lose it" and start driving to the nearest fast-food restaurant, head hunger wins.

Head-hunger eating also provide clues to things you didn't realize were bothering you. When Gail looked back at her vacation, she understood why she ate so many snacks.

On our family trip to Disneyland, I was determined to stay away from snack foods. But two hours into the first day, I'd already eaten a bunch of tortilla chips and a bag of caramel corn. When I thought about head hunger and my "crunchy" foods, I realized I wanted to chew on the costs for admission and the long lines for all of the rides. Together these things added a lot of extra stress to the vacation. —Gail

Bitterness and resentment. Life isn't fair. People cut in line, your family doesn't appreciate you, and someone else gets the promotion you deserve. Do you ever feel angry when people ignore you or don't pay attention to your work? Resentment may cause you to eat out of a desire to "get even" with someone or to prove that people can't tell you what to do.

Have you ever said, "I'll show you" (perhaps under your breath)

Common Head-Hunger Emotions

Anger	Irritation
Stress	Feeling overwhelmed
Resentment	Self-disgust
Frustration	Unfairness
Burnout	Deadlines, pressures
Bitterness	Desire for excitement

---

and proceeded to devour an entire pizza or some other huge quantity of food? Of course, your eating had no effect on those you wanted to punish. It just made you gain weight.

When you hold on to resentment, anger, or hurt for a long time, bitterness creeps in. You may not be aware of these feelings but you can see the results in subtle ways. It took Carol a long time to recognize that her food struggles were related to bitterness over the loss of her marriage.

I have a good job, a nice apartment, and plenty of friends. Some day, I hope to meet a great man and get married again, but for now, I've adjusted to being single. After many years of yo-yo dieting, I'm trying to make better choices about food and eating, but I still struggle with a few bad food habits.

Most days when I get home from work, I head for the cupboard, where I keep a supply of peanut M&Ms. I tell myself, "I'll just have a few of these before dinner," but I often end up eating an entire bag.

I've finally realized that I'm still bitter about the breakup of my marriage. Three years ago, my husband became involved with a female coworker and eventually left me for the other woman. When I come home to my silent apartment, I fight to avoid the memories of happier days when my marriage was strong. I grab the crunchy candies and chew on being single—a lifestyle I never wanted. —Carol

If you have trouble being honest about negative feelings like anger, food may help you avoid facing your emotions. Mary Ann describes her husband as being very critical and demanding. She says, "Whenever I'm talking to him, I try to predict his reaction and plan what to say so he won't get upset. Often it doesn't work and he blows up at me or belittles my opinions. I wish I could be more open, but I can't take the verbal abuse he dumps on me if he doesn't like what I say. So I cautiously tiptoe around the house, often not talking much at all." Mary Ann also sneaks into the kitchen a lot, where food helps shove away her resentment.

Self-disgust. When you've failed many times at losing weight, you may feel angry and disgusted with your own behavior. Marsha has been dieting for years but never seems to make much progress with her goals.

I hate everything—my mirror, my weight and, actually, my life. I've done so many diet programs. Yet, look at me. I'm a blob and I can't seem to change. I even hate the fact that I've screwed up so many times on my weight-loss plans. —Marsha

Out of frustration at herself, Marsha keeps eating more and gaining more weight. Self-directed anger sets up head hunger that leads to more eating, keeping you stuck in the same pattern you want so desperately to fix.

WILL EATING CHANGE MY PROBLEM?

Once you identify what you want to "chew on," ask yourself, "Will eating change this issue?" Will food take away the cause of your stress or alter your child's behavior or eliminate a project deadline? Of course not. Eating might *seem* to fix the problem, because when you eat, you briefly feel calmer or less angry. But after the food is gone, the situation will still be there, often contributing to you eating again. Head-hunger eating simply postpones what you *really* need to do to cope with life.

WHAT TO DO INSTEAD

You don't need a complicated diet plan to manage head-hunger cravings. What you *do* need are quick solutions that provide "buffers" between you and what's causing you to eat. Start by creating a list of things you can do *instead* of eating. Your list might include a few surprisingly simple things, like taking a short walk or listening to music.

These "insteads" won't solve the problem of emotional eating, but they'll allow you time to reflect. Rather than automatically reaching for food, you can think about the cause of your hunger and address the deeper aspects of your emotional needs.

Whatever activity you choose, do it quickly before you change your mind. Don't allow the phrase "a little bit won't hurt me" to weaken your resolve. In many cases, the food *does* hurt you by contributing to more emotional struggles or by harming your self-esteem.

Keep your list available so you can draw on it anytime, especially when you get caught off guard by something unexpected. Use your "insteads" to interrupt the automatic response of eating to take care of your feelings. Here are some ideas to get you started.

- Walk until you feel better, whether that takes ten minutes or an hour.
- Pound on your pillow until your arms are too tired to lift food to your mouth.
- Take several deep breaths. Sigh loudly with each one.
- Clean something you never get around to, like a closet or the "junk" drawer.
- Go to a movie and ignore the concession stand. Focus on the acting and the scenery, then pretend you're a movie critic and write your own review.
- Read something that absorbs you. Plan ahead so you have a couple of good "diversion" books available.
- Wait ten minutes before eating anything. During that time, intentionally do something positive—clean off the top of your

When I want to "chew on" something, instead, I can:

1. Walk, walk, walk. Do something active.

2. Take at least three deep breaths. With each breath, say "I am strong!"

3. Put a stick of gum in my mouth to stop the taste thoughts.

desk, brush your cat, rinse out the coffee pot—or do something nice for somebody else.

After you finish planning things to do instead of eating, select a few that are your favorites. Put these on a separate list to use as your "first response" to emotional hunger. When you start getting a food craving, immediately do at least one of your "first response" items. See an example of a "first response" plan for head hunger, above.

Heart Hunger

Do you ever catch yourself wandering around the house thinking, "I want something to eat, but I don't know what I want?" With heart hunger, you don't usually get a specific food craving—you just start thinking about eating. You might search your cupboards or the refrigerator, unsure of what food sounds good at the moment. You just know you want "something."

When you eventually decide what you "feel" like eating, you very likely will choose something soft, smooth, or creamy. The soothing texture of foods like ice cream or pasta makes them feel satisfying and nurturing. Heart hunger can also push you toward "comfort foods" or foods related to memories of happier times.

Heart hunger shows up in the "empty" or hollow sensations

that make you feel depressed, discouraged, or lonely. You can also blame heart hunger for the desire to eat when you are bored or restless, or when you feel hurt, disappointed, or let down.

Heart hunger can make you want to eat when you're missing something in life or not getting things you want—attention, appreciation, acknowledgment. When life feels awful, self-pity may send you hunting for food to bury your misery.

Do you have trouble resisting sweets or desserts? Many of our happiest memories in life center around times we ate cake, ice cream, or other sweet foods. In some cases, being hooked on sweets might be connected to favorite foods from your childhood, ones that made you feel nurtured, satisfied, and comforted.

Some foods seem to work interchangeably for head and heart hunger, relieving pressure emotions as well as empty ones. These "crossover foods" include things like chocolate and popcorn. A

Common Heart-Hunger Foods

Soft or Creamy	Comfort	Memory
Ice cream	Meatloaf	Casseroles
Pasta, Mexican foods	Mashed potatoes	Homemade desserts
Chocolate	Biscuits and gravy	Fudge, candy
Cinnamon rolls	Pudding, pies	Homemade bread
Cheese	Cakes, cheesecake	Childhood favorites
Eggs	Ethnic foods	Popcorn
Milkshakes	Alcoholic drinks	Mom's cooking

Common Heart-Hunger Emotions and Needs

Sadness	Loneliness
Boredom	Fatigue, illness
Need for attention	Hurt, disappointment
Depression	Discouragement
Restlessness	Hopelessness
Need for love or affection	Lack of meaning

universal "healer," chocolate soothes not only loneliness and sadness but also fury and resentment. With popcorn, the crunchiness meets the chewing needs of head hunger, while the salt and butter entertain your mouth when you feel bored or lonely.

EMPTY EMOTIONS

Instead of the instant craving you get with anger or stress, heart hunger usually creeps in gradually. The feelings tend to be subtle, vague, and hidden, sometimes making it hard to identify what's causing your desire to eat. When you want to escape emotional pain, heart hunger tempts you to use food as a drug. As long as you keep eating, you can avoid thinking about your sadness or loneliness.

Although fatigue and illness aren't emotions, they can tempt you to look for food because you think eating will make you feel better. Sometimes it does—especially if your body needs some nutrition. But lots of times, you don't stop there. You keep eating more, hoping the food will save you from going to bed early or having to take care of yourself in some other way.

Boredom, restlessness. Feeling bored or restless often prompts heart-hunger eating. When you're bored, you want *some-*

thing, but you can't figure out what. Nothing sounds interesting or fun. You turn on the TV, expecting to be entertained, but the shows and even the sporting events disappoint you. It's easy to let food entertain you instead.

At work, Jack spends most of his time making fast-paced decisions and participating in intense discussions. Constantly thinking on his feet, he works at a hectic pace that usually leaves him exhausted at the end of the day. In the evenings, after dinner, Jack often wanders around the house looking for something "sweet" to eat. He never considers himself "bored," yet he obviously feels a vague sense of emptiness after he gets off work.

Eventually Jack realized that his pace in the evenings was just the opposite of his work day. Because he didn't know how to handle this slow, inactive time, he ate out of a subtle form of boredom—the absence of his familiar level of intensity and stress.

Anxiety, doubt, loneliness. Major life changes can shake your confidence by taking you away from the comfort of familiarity and routine. When I moved into a new house a few years ago, I spent weeks getting things unpacked and put away. For me, moving is unsettling. I fret about where to store things and how to organize my dish cupboards and silverware drawers. My insecurity and self-doubt climbed as I worried about how many decorating mistakes I was making.

Soon after the move, I discovered a Dairy Queen a few blocks from my house. Nearly every afternoon, I headed there for an ice cream shake blended with cookies or candy. Eventually I realized what I was doing. When I moved from my old home, I left behind a familiarity that helped me feel safe and secure. In the first months after the move, I routinely used that ice cream treat to fill my empty, unsure feelings. I also gained ten pounds!

Whenever you feel unsure or anxious in life, heart-hunger foods make you feel more secure. People eat their way through all kinds of challenges—moving, getting a divorce, or starting a new job. Food provides comfort any time you face difficult changes in your life.

Feeling invisible. Being overweight can make you feel invisible. People don't want to risk staring at your size, so they gaze past you as if you aren't there. Not being noticed or acknowledged can prompt heart-hunger eating out of feeling alone and isolated.

For much of her childhood and young adult life, Ellen was extremely overweight. She described how feeling trapped in her body contributed to the eating patterns that kept her stuck.

Being a hundred pounds overweight is like walking through life zipped up in a sleeping bag. You can't move, you can't see much, and you feel hot and uncomfortable. People look at you funny, as though you shouldn't be in there. You don't fit in narrow aisles or normal chairs, so you always feel out of place. Living in the sleeping bag is very isolating. You spend a lot of time feeling muffled. Your senses are dulled, making sounds and colors seem a little fuzzy.

What can I do in this sleeping bag? I can eat! That doesn't take much effort so I don't have to move much. Food entertains me and gives me some fun. Besides, it tastes great. And eating is a lot easier than trying to figure out how to get out of this bag. That thought overwhelms me, so I simply stay zipped up. —Ellen

Sometimes you just want it to be "your turn." Instead of doing all the giving, you want someone to nurture and comfort you. To get a hug or have someone hold you would feel so nice. But since there's no one around, you reach for food instead. While you are eating, the food wraps around you and, for a brief moment, makes you feel held and comforted.

What's Empty in My Life?

Whenever you want something to eat but don't know what you want, assume heart hunger is prompting your desire for food. Ask yourself, "What's empty right now? What am I missing in my life? What do I need?"

Perhaps you are alone and wish you had more friends. Maybe difficult times have left you discouraged, sad, or depressed. Or perhaps you're feeling bored or restless because your life lacks challenge or meaning.

Will Eating Change My Situation?

When you start reaching for the first bite of comfort food, ask, "Will eating change my problem?" You'll probably have to admit that eating *does* make things better, at least for a while. Soothing, comforting foods provide a temporary respite from almost any painful feeling. But in the end, nothing changes. Real life is still there, filled with the same empty needs and desires. Like bandaging a skinned knee, food temporarily hides your wounds but it doesn't make them disappear.

What to Do Instead

Just like you did with head hunger, develop a list of heart-hunger "insteads" to draw on whenever you're tempted to eat. With emotions like sadness, you might find comfort in music or reading. If the issue is boredom, learning new hobbies or taking a class might help you cope.

You may notice some overlap with the items from your head-hunger list. For heart-hunger "insteads," you may want to include more things that are nurturing or soothing rather than stimulating activities like exercising. Here are some suggestions.

- Take a warm bath or a hot shower.
- Hug or hold somebody. Consider volunteering at a nursing home or other setting where your hugs would be welcomed.
- Hold or stroke a live animal. If you can't find one, hug a stuffed animal instead.

Is It Head Hunger or Heart Hunger?

How do you recognize it?

Head Hunger
- You know exactly what food you want
- A specific food craving comes on quickly
- You want chewy or crunchy foods (chips, cookies, nuts)
- You want party foods, fun, good-time foods

Heart Hunger:
- You have no specific food in mind
- You want to eat, but don't know what
- You want soft-textured, soothing foods (ice cream, pasta, bread)
- You want nurturing, comfort, or memory foods

What are your emotions?

Head Hunger
- Pressure emotions (anger, frustration, resentment, stress, feeling overwhelmed)
- Intense, instant feelings
- Feeling is present, you want to make it go away
- Emotions are fairly clear, easy to identify
- Food pushes feelings away

Heart Hunger
- Empty emotions (sad, lonely, depressed, bored, restless, needy)
- Missing love, attention, meaning
- Feeling is absent, you want to feel good
- Emotions are vague, hard to identify
- Food buries feelings

- Do something nice for yourself. Get a massage, a facial, or a manicure.
- Light a bunch of candles, especially ones with a fragrance you enjoy.
- Do gardening or other outdoor activities. Appreciate nature.

Possible underlying issues

Head Hunger
- You resent that you can't be honest
- You want to rebel against diet rules
- You hate your weight, you're angry with life
- Eating helps you avoid doing things
- Eating is your only form of fun

Heart Hunger
- You're disappointed with things in life
- You feel like a "nothing," have no self-esteem
- Life didn't turn out like you'd planned
- Eating helps you avoid thinking
- You want to please people, you hope they like you

Questions to ask yourself

Head Hunger
- What do I want to "chew on" in life?
- Will eating change this?
- What can I do instead?

Heart Hunger
- What's empty? What am I missing?
- Will eating change this?
- What can I do instead?

- Give yourself a flower reward. Pick out a specific flower that symbolizes what you need. Or buy a lot of inexpensive flowers and surround yourself with them.
- Listen to a favorite tape or CD. Focus on doing nothing except listening.

Catching Emotional Eating

You may discover that most of your non-hungry eating stems from only one of the two categories, either head hunger or heart hunger. Some people tend to be "stress eaters," whereas others are more likely to eat when they feel bored, depressed, or lonely.

It's also common to experience both types of hunger at once. You might be stressed about a project at work while at the same time you're fighting sadness over a relationship breakup.

Watch for circular patterns with emotional eating. Some people initially eat from head hunger, but after they've "blown it," they shift into heart hunger. Because they feel disappointed with their behavior, they eat more, trying to make up for being helpless and weak around food.

You don't need to lose weight or finish this book before you make changes in your life. You can stop your emotional eating patterns *right now*, as you are reading this, and start a more positive trend in your life.

Anytime you get a food craving, ask yourself, "What's going on?" Then remind yourself that food won't solve your problems. In the chapters ahead, you will learn additional skills for coping with your deeper emotions. But for now, start managing your emotional needs by reaching for your list of "insteads" rather than automatically grabbing something to eat.

CHAPTER FOUR

Rebuilding Self-Esteem

ON THE MORNING LIZ WORE her new suit to work, she was determined to look great. She spent extra time on her hair and makeup, and even searched out a pair of hose with no runs. The suit was beautiful—dark navy with a subtle pinstripe. The double-breasted jacket and slim, calf-length skirt fit nicely.

As she walked down the hall toward her office, Liz waited for someone to notice how terrific she looked. It didn't take long. Dorothy, a fashion-conscious manager from accounting, paused as she met Liz. "Nice suit," she said. Then her eyes slid downward and she added, "But those shoes don't seem to work with it. Maybe a pair of smooth black pumps would help pull it together."

Liz choked out a quick "thank you," then stumbled toward her office, closed the door, and burst into tears. Once again, she had screwed up. "Why can't I ever get it right?" she wondered. "I try so hard to dress like a sharp, professional woman, but I've failed at it again." Throughout the rest of the day, she kept feeling the sting of Dorothy's words. When she finally got home, Liz hung the suit in her closet and never wore it again.

When Liz looked back on that day, she told me, "I'm still both-ered by my reaction. I wish I'd had a better response—some snappy comeback that would have let me ignore Dorothy's words. But I got caught off guard by her comment. I immediately concluded she must be right and that something was wrong with *me!*"

How many times have you done this? Instead of evaluating whether a criticism is true, you assume it's accurate and that you are at fault. So when someone makes a snide comment about your looks or your abilities, you add it to your list of personal defects. Eventually, these negative images can undermine your entire sense of identity.

As you separate your food cravings into head and heart hunger, you'll begin to see places where low self-esteem keeps you from taking action. In this chapter, you will learn how to rebuild a weak self-image and create a new belief system about yourself. You'll dis-cover how to rebound quickly and rebuild your self-esteem when something zaps it away. As you change your inner picture of who you are, you'll become much more confident about your ability to manage your weight.

Often, a lack of self-esteem is at the core of emotional eating. It also affects your belief about whether or not you can change. When you strengthen your self-esteem, you improve your success with emotional eating and motivation as well as your ability to stay on a diet plan.

The Power of Self-Esteem

Very simply, self-esteem is *feeling good about yourself.* People with high self-esteem tend to exude confidence, feel comfortable with their bodies, and see themselves as valuable. Now that doesn't sound so hard, does it? Then why do so many people, particularly women, rate low self-esteem as their number-one barrier to success in nearly all aspects of life?

Most of the women at my clinic listed "Improve how I feel about myself" as one of their top reasons for wanting to lose weight. Only "health issues" consistently ranked higher than self-esteem. But which comes first—being overweight or having low self-esteem? Actually, it doesn't matter. The real issue is the vicious circle that results when these two problems keep fueling each other.

Self-esteem gets tied to weight struggles because *food makes you feel good!* When a grueling experience devastates your confidence and self-trust, food soothes the pain. It gives you the courage to face the world again.

Of course, at the same time, overeating destroys self-esteem by making you feel disgusted and frustrated. Like Liz, you may develop a belief that "something's wrong with me." When you eat to cope with a poor self-image, you gain more weight, which ultimately pulls your self-esteem even lower.

It's hard to follow through with an action plan when you've lost confidence in yourself. In fact, if you've gained a lot of weight, low self-esteem can even damage your resolve to stay on a weight-loss program. How do you reconstruct your self-esteem when you've slid so far down?

Here's the good news. Regardless of your current life situation, you can still find your inner spirit and rebuild your self-esteem. And it won't take years to accomplish. By making a few simple changes in your self-talk and your internal beliefs, you can improve your self-esteem almost immediately.

SEE YOUR POTENTIAL

Imagine you're walking through a forest when you spot a piece of wood nearly hidden in a pile of leaves. As you study the layers of moss and caked-on dirt that cover it, you can't see any beauty in this scrap of wood and you question whether it has any value.

But something compels you to pick it up and carry it home. In your workshop, you carefully scrape off the dirt, then begin sanding and polishing your wood. To your astonishment, you uncover a deep grain filled with rich, beautiful colors.

As you continue restoring the wood, you start planning how you could use it for some special purpose. Your excitement builds as you envision creating a unique picture frame or a graceful table leg. There's no doubt in your mind that this piece of wood has great value.

You are this piece of wood. Even when painful layers such as your weight or other burdens cover your beauty, the real *you* never disappears. Your value as a person doesn't change because of what you look like or what happens to you. Underneath your discouragement and low self-esteem, you are still *you*, as strong and vibrant as ever.

CREATE A NEW RESPONSE

Difficult events in your life don't ruin your self-esteem—it's what you *tell yourself* about those events that does the damage. Dorothy's comments didn't change the suit, but Liz told herself they did. Instead of walking proudly in her new clothes, she suddenly felt embarrassed to have anyone see her. She also concluded that because she didn't know how to dress right, it was her own fault Dorothy said those hurtful things.

It never occurred to her to flip the words around and tell herself, "I *know* I look fabulous today. In fact, I would look great in this suit even if I was barefoot!" What if she could have secretly laughed at Dorothy's "tacky" behavior and concluded that something was wrong with *her*, not Liz? Or perhaps she could have acted pleased and asked Dorothy for advice on shoes, even inviting her to go shopping together sometime.

Had she used any of these responses, Liz would have continued to feel confident about her appearance. But to do this, *she needed to feel better about herself to begin with.* Having strong self-esteem gives you the courage to face difficult comments and situations without crumbling.

Think back to the example of the piece of wood. You may have to scrape off a few old beliefs and habits, but you *can* build self-esteem that remains strong, no matter what happens in your life. Soon, your renewed self-image will add power to your efforts for conquering emotional eating and managing your weight.

Self-esteem can be approached in a variety of ways. In this book, I have divided it into three simple categories:

• How you *see* yourself and how you think others see you.
• What you *say* to yourself.
• What you *believe* about yourself, including your confidence and your value.

First, we'll study each area separately, and you'll learn skills and tricks for altering your old patterns. Then I'll show you how to merge these three concepts into powerful self-esteem that will carry you through all of life's events—including insensitive comments about your shoes!

How You See Yourself

Even though you try to avoid it, sometimes you can't help comparing yourself to other people. There's always someone who is thinner, smarter, more attractive, or more talented than you are. Advertisements add to this by portraying smooth complexions, silky hair, and shapely legs or "washboard" abs. And the people shown on billboards or in movies and TV shows certainly don't look like you.

How do you respond to these images? Can you ignore them and appreciate your own lumpy body for what it is? Or do these images of perfection remind you of all of the areas where you think you're lacking?

How you see yourself encompasses not only your physical appearance, but your competence, your intelligence, and your life skills. If you think about yourself right now, do you picture a confident, slender, capable person? Or do you instantly see someone who is fat, unattractive, or dumpy? What about clumsy or awkward? Do you ever label yourself as lazy, unproductive, or unsuccessful?

When you hold a negative view of yourself, you tend to match it by how you live. Any time you see yourself as "weak" around food, you overeat. If your primary mental picture of yourself is a "fat slob," your efforts to lose weight will usually fail.

To change the way you "see" yourself, you have to create different images. I'm not suggesting you pretend you're thin when you aren't. But you can change the way you view your actions and your potential. Instead of seeing yourself as a failure, build an image of forward movement and progress. Rather than dwelling on failures, notice those areas in which you're successful.

SMALL WINS

Janet was frustrated with her "wasted" day. As she recalled her struggles, I suggested she start at the beginning and describe the entire day as she remembered it.

Yesterday was an awful day! I ate too much, I didn't exercise, I yelled at the kids, and I burned the dinner. Lately, every day seems to be the same way—I have good intentions, but most of the time I don't follow through with any of them.

I guess I did a few things right. I cooked oatmeal for my eight-year-old, who loves it. I ran out the door to give my husband the project book he'd forgotten on the kitchen table. Then I sat on the patio with my coffee and did deep-breathing exercises while I appreciated the fresh morning air.

When I got to my job at the store, I listened to an employee who had a sick child. I drank four glasses of water by noon, made a telephone call to a depressed friend, called my husband for an update on his stressful meeting, and wrote an outline for my church women's class. I ate cottage cheese and an apple for lunch. When I got home, I picked up Jenny's room to surprise her, let my husband watch TV without interruption for an hour, and trimmed off the overcooked areas of the casserole so my family wouldn't have to eat them.

At this point in Janet's story, I interrupted her. "Wait a minute. I'm amazed at what a wonderful, caring, successful day you had! A minute ago, you had a whole list of things that went wrong. Where are they in this day?" Janet thought and then quietly admitted, "I can't remember any of them!"

It's easy to get hung up on the "bad" things that happen and see only your failures. To change this pattern, train yourself to do the opposite and focus on the positive things or "small wins" instead of minor slip-ups.

Start noticing your small wins by writing down all the good things that happen in a day. Make note of your actions as well as the outcomes that result. Your list can include anything that makes you feel productive, happy, or successful.

In the past, you may have followed a diet plan that had you write down everything you eat. Not this time! For your small wins list, ignore any food struggles and instead record only positive eating events or healthy foods. Leave out the doughnuts you had this morning but list the apple you ate at lunch. You can skip writing down the candy bar you ate on the way home, but be sure to include the salad you had at dinner.

At the end of the day, commend yourself for all your accomplishments. Keep this up for at least a week, perhaps even several months. Each night, read your list and notice how it affects your attitude. Within even a few days, you'll start seeing yourself as a "success" instead of a "failure."

AT MY BEST...

What are you like when you're living and performing at your best? Think about times when you were at a healthy weight or were exercising regularly. Recall jobs or school years when you were doing great work. Picture your best friendships or the excitement of being in love.

Remember days when you've felt confident, strong, capable, and able to face challenges head on. Even if it's been years ago, think of times when you were truly at your best, physically as well as mentally and emotionally.

In a notebook or on a piece of paper, write *"At my best, here's how I am..."*

Then write down every descriptive word and phrase you can think of that portrays how you act, look, feel, or live when you are at your best. When you finish, read your list and notice the energy and enthusiasm it generates.

Here's an example of this exercise done by Rita, a client in my weight-loss clinic.

At my best, here's how I am:
• Energetic, bouncy, smile a lot, twinkly eyes.
• Laugh easily, tell jokes, feel good physically.

- Grounded, centered, confident about my abilities.
- Productive, hard worker, accomplish a lot.
- Blend well with people, relate easily, enjoy my friends.
- Hug and cuddle my husband a lot, encourage sex and intimacy.
- Connected spiritually, cultivate my faith, attend church regularly.
- Physically strong, fit, flexible, play tennis and golf.

Rita told me she loves reading her list because it reminds her to live what she wrote. She says, "Whenever I start feeling down on myself, instead of looking for cheesecake or some other nurturing food, I review my list. It almost immediately pulls me out of the dumps and helps me skip the eating part."

Save your list and read it often, especially when your self-esteem droops. By recalling your favorite personality traits, you remember who you really are as a person. This positive vision becomes critical to the self-esteem component of how you "see" yourself.

What You Say to Yourself

For a number of years, Vicki struggled with weight gain fueled by marriage problems, a failed secretarial business, and a move from New York to Arizona that took her away from her friends and family. During the time she was steadily gaining weight, she constantly blamed herself. In her head, she would say things like, "You are such a failure. You got yourself into this mess, so you deserve the problems you're having right now."

The more she focused on her helplessness, the more she ate. At her highest weight of three hundred and twenty pounds, Vicki was so miserable she could barely look at herself in the mirror. Every day, she reminded herself how awful she was and how she would never be able to change.

When Vicki made plans to visit her family back in New York, she dreaded the trip for weeks. Because of her weight, she knew she wasn't going fit into the airline seat easily. Once she boarded the plane, she maneuvered herself into the space by the window and tried to take up as little room as possible.

Minutes later, she heard a loud male voice announce to a flight attendant, "I'm sorry, but you'll have to reassign me to another seat! This lady is taking up so much room, I couldn't possibly fit comfortably in the same row as her." This humiliation only added to the negative phrases Vicki was already mentally rehearsing. Since the seat next to her remained empty during the flight, no one saw the tears that flowed down her cheeks.

About an hour into the flight, Vicki felt a hand on her shoulder. When she raised her head, she looked into the kind face of a flight attendant, who leaned over to speak close to her ear. "I apologize for that insensitive man. Don't let him ruin your day! You are a valuable person and don't ever tell yourself that you aren't!"

Vicki was stunned. No one had ever said she was a valuable person! She also realized that everything she'd been telling herself was the exact opposite. At that moment, Vicki straightened her shoulders and made a decision. She was *valuable*. And because of that, she was going to start living like a valuable person.

During the remainder of the flight, she began telling herself things like, "You are a beautiful woman. You are strong and capable. You can do anything you want in life." She also vowed she would *never* face a situation like that again.

After that turning point, Vicki joined a new weight-loss program and subsequently lost one hundred and sixty-five pounds. In addition to maintaining a healthy weight herself, Vicki now mentors other overweight women. Her goal is to help them achieve weight-loss success, partly by changing what they say to themselves.

ELIMINATE "JUNK TALK"

What you say to yourself can make or break nearly everything you do. You are what you think you are. Phrases like "I can't do anything right" or "I'm such a failure" certainly don't inspire you to change your patterns. "Junk talk" serves no purpose in your life. In fact, devaluing statements and half-truths usually pull you further into despair.

The opposite is also true. Practice saying to yourself "Come on, you can do anything!" You'll be amazed at how that phrase helps you stay on target with your goals. Vicki discovered that telling herself "I am a valuable person" made a significant difference in her ability to manage her weight.

In his self-esteem training workshops, Jack Canfield, coauthor of the *Chicken Soup for the Soul* series, teaches a unique way to change self-talk. He encourages participants to counter any negative messages by saying, "No matter what you say or do to me, I am still a worthwhile person!"

To reinforce this belief, he hurls insults at the class members, yelling things like "you're fat" or "you're ugly." The students have to respond by shouting back the "worthwhile person" line. When you say this phrase over and over, you mentally contradict "cutdown" messages that previously would have undermined your self-esteem.

CHANGE YOUR VOCABULARY

If you've struggled with your weight for a long time, you may have adopted some common "dieting phrases" to describe your behavior. As part of improving your self-esteem, evaluate what you say to yourself when you slip off your plan or lose motivation. Eliminate the phrases that pull you down by changing them to a more positive message. Here are a few important ways to change your vocabulary.

"I blew it." Whenever you say "I blew it" in response to an eating slip-up, you give yourself a message of discouragement and failure. Those words also prompt you to conclude, "Since I blew it anyway, I might as well continue to eat. I'll start my diet over tomorrow." Soon a minor eating slip-up becomes a major food binge. Not only does one mistake ruin your current plan, it also negates your previous weight-loss efforts.

Beverly described how she would use an eating binge to punish herself for minor infractions on her diet plan. She said, "It's like I back my car into a post, but instead of quickly assessing the damage and driving away, I decide that one dent isn't enough. So I keep slamming my car backward into the post over and over to pay for my first mistake."

Practice viewing a slip-up as a minor event, not a crisis. If you eat something that's not on your plan, don't beat yourself with harsh, punishing words like "I blew it." Instead, label the incident as a "pause" in your program. This gentle word doesn't make detrimental references to your personality or your ability to accomplish a goal. Simply say, "I had a brief pause, but now I'm back on track." Then let go of the behaviors in your "pause" and move on.

"I cheated." You can't cheat with food! It's impossible. You can cheat on your taxes or perhaps on your partner, but you can't cheat on your diet. The word cheat refers to something illegal or immoral, and food is neither of these.

Stop using the word "cheat" when you refer to any aspect of your eating plan. Instead, refer to your behavior as a "choice." If you eat a cookie that wasn't on your diet, say, "I chose to eat a cookie today." Maybe you wish you hadn't, but either way, you made a *choice* about eating it.

In the same way, stop referring to yourself as "good" or "bad," based on what you ate. Since food is not a moral issue, you can't apply behavioral codes to what you do with it. Again, use the word "choice" when you describe your compliance with a food plan. Some days you make great choices, other days you don't do as well. By referring to your actions as a choice, you eliminate the punishing self-message that says you were "bad."

REFRAME THE SITUATION

When you reframe an event or a thought, you view it from a different perspective. The word "reframing" simply refers to changing the way you think or speak about something. For example, if it rained on the day you were planning a picnic, you could reframe your disappointment by saying, "This is great! Now I don't have to worry about getting bugs or dust in my food." Or you could view the rain as a welcome excuse to curl up in your favorite chair with a good book.

When you reframe a situation or an idea, you don't deny its existence, you simply take a fresh view toward it and invent a new message. Whenever an old thought hooks you, turn it into a positive statement by saying, "That's not true! Actually...", then fill in the sentence with a new ending.

When you reframe something, you simply take the picture from a different angle. By reframing what you say to yourself, you can become an encouraging, positive voice instead of putting yourself down. In the long run, you'll achieve much better results than when you hold on to your old negative viewpoints.

Banish the beating stick. Suppose you went to a party and overate—a lot! What do you say to yourself on the way home? If you mentally beat yourself up for how you ate, by the time you get home, your self-esteem will be in the toilet. But by reframing the evening's events, you can understand what happened and plan how to manage that situation differently next time.

Reframe the Situation

Old phrase	That's not true! Actually...
• I can't do anything right.	• I do lots of things extremely well.
• I've never been able to maintain my weight.	• I've learned many tools that maintain my weight give me the ability
• I'm such a failure.	• I'm a success at many things. For example: _____.

First, look beyond what you ate and assess which emotions or needs were affecting you. Were you feeling insecure around the other people at the event? Did a desire to relax and have fun become a higher priority than healthy eating? By figuring out what contributed to an evening of emotional eating, you can be much kinder in what you say to yourself.

As you become skilled at reframing, you won't find it necessary to berate yourself for your struggles. In fact, you might as well get rid of the mental stick you use to beat yourself up. Hold a small ceremony to destroy your "beating stick" and affirm that you'll never use it again.

Find a tree branch or a small piece of wood that looks like a "beating stick" to you. Sit on a hillside or in front of your fireplace and hold your "stick" tightly. Close your eyes and remember all the things you've said to yourself as you've hammered away with that stick. Recall saying things like "You can't ever stay on a diet" or "You've blown it again."

Decide that you'll no longer use that stick to punish your weaknesses around food, exercise, or other behaviors in your life. Then get rid of your beating stick by burning it or throwing it far away.

As you turn from your ceremony, remind yourself the stick is totally gone and you will never pick it up again.

When you review your eating behaviors, practice using a kind, gentle voice for your self-talk. Learn from your struggles, then erase your mental blackboard and let them go. Use a reframing such as "I ate it; I'm over it; I'm doing better now." Then move forward, determined to manage your eating in healthier ways in the future.

Compliment the complimenter. When someone compliments you, what do you say to yourself and to the other person? It's easy to respond with, "Thanks for telling me I look nice, but my hair looks awful today." Or perhaps you explain why the compliment is false, saying, "Oh, but this dress is so old and it makes me look fat."

When you respond to a compliment, be careful about making other people "wrong" by arguing with their observation. Instead, learn to receive compliments without squirming because you don't believe the words are true.

If getting a compliment makes you uncomfortable, work at turning it around by validating the person who gave it. This technique takes a little practice but it will revolutionize the way you handle praise. Whenever someone pays you a compliment, acknowledge it, then give back the "gift of appreciation."

Suppose a friend says, "You look great today. I just love that dress." Here's how you might respond. "Wow! It's so nice of you to say something. I can't tell you how much it means to hear those words. In fact, you just made my day by saying that. Thank you."

This method goes beyond accepting a compliment graciously. It actually switches the focus to the other person and helps you avoid feeling self-conscious or embarrassed by the attention. In using this technique, you present a gift to the person who gave you the compliment.

What You Believe

Changing what you "see" and what you "say" will certainly improve your self-esteem. But at the same time, if you hold on to your old beliefs, your self-confidence stays weak. Beliefs aren't always obvious, yet in their subtle ways, they affect many of your results.

Andrea was having a difficult time with her twelve-year-old son. The school was threatening to expel him for his consistent behavioral problems. He had no close friends, and at home, he stayed in his room for hours. Finally, Andrea contacted a well-known child psychologist to see if he could determine what was wrong with her son and help him improve his behavior.

When they arrived for their initial counseling session, the therapist requested to first meet with the son alone. He took the boy into his office and spent ten minutes teaching him magic tricks. Then the therapist instructed him to stand in front of a mirror in the outer room and practice the tricks he'd been taught.

For the remaining forty minutes, the therapist met with the boy's mother. This went on for many weeks. The therapist would spend ten minutes teaching the boy magic, then send him out to practice while Andrea had her session.

After a couple of months, the boy's behavior began to change. He came out of his room a lot more and he started doing magic tricks for his family and grandparents. At school, his behavior improved as he became somewhat of an entertainer. His stronger self-confidence also helped him develop a new set of friends.

Andrea remained skeptical. One week she complained to the therapist that he never talked with her son about his "problems." When the therapist asked how her son seemed to be doing, she described how his behavior had completely turned around at school and his grades had improved. She also mentioned his new friends and the way he participated in family events at home.

The therapist responded, "Your son didn't believe he was capable of doing anything worthwhile. He needed to build confidence in himself and his own personality. Learning magic tricks proved to him that he's a smart, capable human being. Simply building his self-esteem made all the difference in his behavior."

KICK YOUR OLD BELIEFS

When you tell yourself something over a long time, eventually you don't remember it being any other way. If you felt awkward or clumsy as a child, you may have told yourself you are too uncoordinated to participate in sports. As an adult, these old beliefs can prevent you from learning to play tennis or trying in-line skating or golf.

Do you secretly believe you'll always gain back the weight you lose, regardless of which diet plan you go on? If so, your behavior will follow the same line as your thoughts, eliminating any chance of successfully managing your weight.

You may need to dismantle your flawed beliefs and replace them with new messages. Even if something was true in the past, it doesn't have to stay that way forever. See if you still hold on to some of these old beliefs.

"I have no willpower!" Have you convinced yourself that you don't have any willpower? What a great excuse for overeating! Since you don't have any willpower, it's not your fault you give in to pastries or your mom's chocolate cake. If you believe you are powerless around food because you have no willpower, you create a self-fulfilling prophecy.

Willpower is a myth. It's not something you either have or don't have. Instead, your ability to resist a food temptation comes from believing you can do it. Instead of assuming you don't have willpower, go back to the concept of making choices.

Sometimes you might choose to eat because the food meets an emotional need or you miss a particular taste or texture. But you are also capable of choosing to NOT eat. To do this successfully, look beyond your food craving and determine how else you could meet your needs at that moment.

"I'm a compulsive overeater!" Do you ever start eating, then feel like you absolutely can't stop? What about when you feel "out of control" and stuff yourself with everything in sight? If you feel like you can't stop eating, you may assume you're a compulsive overeater.

In truth, you probably don't fit the "compulsive" definition at all. The word "compulsive" refers to an uncontrolled, urgent desire that cannot be stopped voluntarily. People diagnosed with obsessive–compulsive disorders experience this as a frightening behavioral struggle.

Instead, you're probably an *impulsive overeater*. With this pattern, you react on "impulse" to something that makes you desire food or want to keep eating. Seeing or smelling food can prompt an impulsive eating response. So can feelings of stress, frustration, or sadness. Any time you experience an uncomfortable emotion, you may impulsively react by using food to make the feelings go away.

Even though you may feel like you can't stop yourself, you *can* control impulsive eating. When you're on a tight budget, you can usually talk yourself out of impulsively buying an expensive item. In the same way, you can train yourself to manage impulses differently around food. For example, you could cope with a stressful event by taking a walk instead of impulsively grabbing something to eat.

Whenever you're tempted to label yourself as a "compulsive eater," remind yourself that this simply isn't true. Then see if you can determine which emotions or needs are promoting your impulsive reaction. Instead of allowing your impulses around food to control your life, convince yourself that *you* are in charge of your own actions.

"I'm nobody!" Do you often feel like you don't count or that you aren't important? At the heart of self-esteem lies your ability to view yourself as a valuable, important human being, deserving of respect. So whenever you slide into thinking you're "nobody," you weaken your self-esteem.

Your true value doesn't come from the wonderful things you do, the children you raise, or the business you run. You are valuable *because you exist.* From the moment you entered this earth as an infant, you became an asset to the world.

It's easy to lose sight of your real value and believe that your worth is based on how much you weigh or how you look. This might be true if you were a Hollywood star, a fashion model, or a star athlete. But most likely you aren't. You're probably a hard-working person who is dedicated to making a decent living and caring for the people in your life.

To see your value differently, picture yourself down on your knees in front of a small child. As you look this child in the eye, you might say, "The fact that you ate candy before dinner or broke your toy doesn't change who you are. You are still valuable regardless of what you did."

Make an effort to treat yourself with the same tenderness and respect as you would that child. Hold your head up high and repeatedly tell yourself, "I'm important, I'm valuable, I count in this world."

Here's another way to remind yourself of your value. Each night before you go to bed, talk to yourself out loud in front of a mirror. Review your day by listing all the things you appreciate about yourself. Recall ways you demonstrated your inner value by showing kindness, sensitivity, or caring toward somebody else.

Finish by saying "I love you" to yourself in the mirror. You may feel silly doing this, but within a short time, you'll see your value differently. When you believe in yourself based on *who you are inside*, you strengthen your self-confidence in all aspects of your life.

FIND SUCCESS SOMEWHERE

When you get overwhelmed, everything can seem to go wrong at the same time. Because work has been crazy for weeks, your exercise plan falls apart. Your house is a disaster and you keep ordering pizza because you can't get to the grocery store. On top of everything else, your car breaks down and you don't know where you'll get the money to fix it.

During times like this, figure out how to find "success somewhere," by making progress in one area of your life. Choose a place to start and pick one task you *know* you can accomplish. For example, maybe you could get back to your exercise program by doing a ten-minute walk after you get home from work. That small success motivates you to eat something healthy for dinner. Suddenly you feel stronger about planning changes at work that will help cut your stress.

Don't assume you need to fix all areas of your life at once. You just need to get *one* thing to work. One tiny success will soon overflow into other areas, helping you improve them as well. If you have a day when nothing goes right, simply break the pattern. Choose one small activity or task you know you can do well, then do it.

Once you finish, commend yourself mentally, then move on to another goal. Each time you successfully complete a task, you reinforce a belief that you can do more. After you achieve a few small successes, you'll find it easier to sustain momentum with your other goals.

LIST YOUR STRENGTHS

On difficult days, when you don't feel very strong, you may need to remind yourself that you *really are* competent or successful. To help you do this, build a list of what is "almost true" about yourself. In your notebook or on a piece of paper write: *"My strengths: What I am even if I don't always believe it or do it."*

Then create a list of your best strengths, using these three categories: 1) physical attributes; 2) skills and abilities; 3) personality traits. Stretch your mental self-image as much as you can to make your list match the way you are deep inside, even if you don't always feel that way. Include words like "good weight" or "physically fit" even if right now your weight is up and you haven't exercised in a while. You will be drawing on this list for years to come, so along with your current strengths, include ones you will return to in the future.

Don't discount items on your list by saying, "I'm not really that attractive (kind, creative)." Instead, hold tightly to the belief that you *are* attractive, kind, or creative, even during times when you don't feel or act that way. For example, even on a day when you yell at another driver or snap at a coworker, you still are a kind and considerate person.

Megan is a graphic artist who works as a marketing director at a large company. She struggles with the demands of a challenging job as well as keeping balance in her home life with a husband and two young children. Over the last few years, a weight gain of almost forty pounds has greatly affected her self-esteem.

Building her list wasn't easy for Megan because, at that moment, she didn't see herself as attractive or highly competent. Yet when she dug into her memories of how her life had been in

Megan's Strengths

1. Physical attributes

Healthy, good weight, athletic, strong, attractive, pretty, appealing, sexy, nice eyes, pretty hair, nice body, active, energetic, bouncy

2. Skills and abilities

Intelligent, knowledgeable, quick learner, skilled, competent, organized, capable, creative, detail oriented, thorough, good worker, quick thinker, decisive, confident, domestic—cook, clean, sew, do crafts, good parent

3. Personality traits

Sensitive, intuitive, thoughtful, caring, kind, gentle, patient, loving, sweet, pleasant, assertive, strong, fun, enjoyable to be with

---

times past, she realized her skills and strengths were still there, even if she wasn't using them right now. See Megan's list, above.

As you create your own list, fill it with past strengths as well as your current ones. Over the next few weeks, read your list often. You might even memorize it so you can easily recite it while driving or doing other activities. Any time you struggle with weak self-esteem or you doubt your own abilities, use your strength list to renew your confidence and belief in yourself.

Jeff worked at a busy architectural firm that usually had extremely tight project deadlines. When he was feeling the intensity of finishing a work proposal, he would snack continually through the afternoon. Jeff often felt insecure around the other engineers, and he knew he was using food to increase his confidence in his own work.

After completing his list of strengths, Jeff made several copies of it and carried one with him everywhere. His most powerful benefit came when he realized he could use it to build his confidence for the day.

I wrote my strengths on a card and kept it on the visor in my car. Every morning on the drive to work, I rehearsed the list, often embellishing it with references to my current situation. I'd remind myself that I am organized and creative and that those skills were going to pull me through the demanding project I had to face that day. Once I started feeling stronger about my work skills and my capabilities, I realized I didn't need my afternoon snacks to help me believe I could do my job well. —Jeff

Your New Self

Now it's time to blend the components of self-esteem into a total picture. Start each day by creating an image of yourself as a successful person. In a mirror, practice looking past the imperfections you see and simply love yourself. Read your description of "At my best, here's how I am" whenever you need a reminder of who you *really* are.

When you face difficult events or situations, remind yourself that *you are a worthwhile person*, regardless of what others say or do. Build small successes into your day, adding to your belief that you are capable of accomplishing your goals. Review your list of strengths regularly, always reminding yourself they are accurate, even on days when you don't use them.

Self-esteem doesn't happen by default. To have great self-esteem, you have to build it from the ground up, then nurture it daily to keep it strong. So regularly practice the techniques you've learned in this chapter. Don't allow yourself to slide back into your old ways of thinking or your previous beliefs about yourself as a person.

LIVE "AS IF"

Researchers have long known that acting "as if" you have a skill or a feeling eventually contributes to its coming true. Public speakers are taught to address their audience "as if" they feel totally confident and have no stage fright whatsoever. Most speakers discover that after doing this just a few times, it becomes true.

In a study done many years ago, two groups of people who were depressed agreed to take walks as part of an experiment. The people in one group were told to walk for twenty minutes each day. The others were told the same thing, but with one added instruction. Regardless of how depressed they felt, during their walk they were to hold their head high and walk with a spirited step "as if" they felt great. By the end of the study, nearly all the participants from the "as if" group reported a significant decrease in their feelings of depression and hopelessness.

You don't have to wait until "some day" to have self-esteem. You can build your confidence and self-image by acting "as if" you already feel good about yourself. Even if you don't completely believe it, use powerful and convincing self-talk to reinforce your capabilities and your delightful personality.

When you get dressed each day, look in the mirror and say, "I look great!" It doesn't matter if you're wearing a baggy dress and worn shoes. *Pretend!* Imagine how you would talk to others, do your work, and raise your children if you truly felt great about yourself. Then live out of that internal picture, acting "as if" those things were true.

Taking this approach doesn't mean you can put your head in the sand or ignore the realities of life. It just helps you develop a new attitude about what's already there. At the same time, it also gives you hope that things can get better. After a month or so of living "as if" you are confident and strong about yourself, you'll be amazed at how well you match this image.

When Self-Esteem Falters

You've learned a lot of techniques for building self-esteem. Now you need to practice, rehearse, and memorize the concepts you've learned. But despite all your efforts at self-talk and building new beliefs, you will probably still experience times when your power fizzles.

A relationship breakup or a tongue-lashing from your boss might be a little too much for your fragile self-esteem skills. Instead of making a snappy comeback or walking tall, you sink into despair. When your old "I'm no good" messages come rushing back, how do you rebound and get your self-esteem to work again?

GET LOGICAL

Your brain has a logical side and an emotional side. These two different thought patterns constantly battle for top position. The logic side firmly but gently reminds you of things like how to use the phrase "At my best, here's how I am." Logical concepts guide you through challenges such as coping with the temptation to overeat. They also help you believe in yourself and your ability to make life work.

When your emotional side controls your thoughts, you say things like "I can't do this. I'll never be successful. It's hopeless." Then you further weaken your self-esteem by adding a few demeaning words like stupid, fat, or ugly. When you go through a hard time and totally mess up your plan, your emotional side celebrates. It knows you are about to give in and believe what it's telling you. To counteract this side of your thinking and salvage your self-esteem, you must force yourself to listen to the logical side.

Pull out your notebook or the pieces of paper on which you've recorded the exercises in this chapter. Read all your lists, from your "small wins" and "At my best" to your "list of strengths." Look for the truth in a challenging situation and push aside the emotional whining that threatens to pull you down. Consciously push yourself into more logical thoughts until you can rebound and see things in a healthier, more positive light.

I'm not saying you'll never feel pain or hurt. Acknowledging your feelings and needs remains an important part of your self-esteem recovery. But along with your tears or your anger, ask your logical side to help you be more rational and separate a negative event from how you see yourself.

PRACTICE INSTANT SELF-ESTEEM

Any time you struggle to remember your skills, use this quick exercise to instantly boost your self-esteem. Read these three phrases in rapid succession, out loud if possible:

I have sparkling eyes, I have a warm smile, and I'm going to make it!

Repeat the entire sequence of phrases several times. You will be amazed at how it instantly improves your mood. When you say "I have sparkling eyes" several times in a row, your brain picks up the message and actually makes your eyes sparkle.

You can vary the last phrase to match situations such as conducting a meeting, going on a job interview, or preparing for a date. Just substitute words like "I'm going to be great" or "I'm going to do my absolute best."

———

Self-esteem is an ongoing project. But now you know how to create and reinforce it, so you can keep it strong through nearly every situation that comes along. Remember, self-esteem isn't based on what happens to you, but on what you tell yourself about what happens. Keep building your inner strength, and you'll become a much better friend and support to yourself.

CHAPTER FIVE

What Do I Feel?

REMEMBER HOW EASILY YOUR emotions came when you were a child? You rolled around on the floor when you laughed and you never worried about whether you looked silly. When you fell and skinned your knee, you wailed loudly and cried hot tears. You screamed in anger when your brother threw your favorite doll in the mud. Most of the time, you never questioned whether these emotions made sense—you just expressed what you felt.

Then you began to grow up. You learned to tone down your outbursts and stifle your giggles. When you slammed a drawer on your finger, you shook off the pain and swallowed your tears. Instead of hitting your brother, you ignored his teasing and walked away.

Some of this was necessary. In the adult world, you can't always show everything you feel. But sometimes, you end up pushing your emotions away too far. In your efforts to moderate your feelings, you can lose touch with how they work.

Maybe you try hard to stay "in control" and never show how you feel. So when you get angry at your boss, you don't say anything. You may not be able to remember the last time you cried.

Many days, you probably don't feel anything except stressed or tired, neither of which is an emotion.

But not thinking about feelings doesn't mean you don't have them. Emotions are normal. If you refuse to acknowledge them, you have to figure out how to keep them hidden. So instead of dealing with your feelings, you grab something to eat and push them away.

To stop these eating patterns, you may have to take the lid off your buried emotions. I'm not suggesting you eliminate all restraint when showing your feelings. Social etiquette dictates that you can't cry in the middle of a staff meeting or slam your desk drawers when you get angry. But if you are determined to manage emotional eating, you can't keep shoving your feelings away.

Living in an emotionally healthy way involves being able to access the entire range of your emotions. You can't choose to allow only happy thoughts and ignore feelings of sadness or frustration. Even though it's difficult, you must be able to genuinely and accurately express *all* of your feelings.

Exploring your emotions may help you uncover thoughts and experiences you'd forgotten about. As you rediscover positive feelings like joy, relief, or peace, you will also find the courage to face emotions that feel a little uncomfortable.

In Step Two of conquering emotional eating, you'll be asking yourself "What do I feel?" In the next chapter, you'll learn how to express your emotions in healthy and satisfying ways. But for now, just work on noticing and labeling your feelings.

Family Influence on Emotions

Think about how emotions were handled during your growing-up years. Were you allowed to cry? How about having temper tantrums or showing anger? Were you ever stopped in the middle of having fun because you were "too loud" or "too silly"?

Most families operate with unspoken but definite rules about how to feel and express emotions. These "rules" help you determine what is acceptable and what feelings you can never show.

In our home, Mom often told us, "Stop crying or I'll give you something to cry about." I learned very young that it's not ladylike to lose your temper and that I had to "quit being so silly." The worst rule was having to apologize for things that I wasn't sorry about! —Jennifer

Along with your family rules, you also learned what happened when you expressed certain feelings. Did you ever experience pain or sadness or anger and get told your feelings were "wrong"? Maybe you were scolded for whining or chided with "You shouldn't feel that way," or "That's not how you really feel." But this didn't make sense to you, because at the same you were being told not to feel, you definitely felt something.

A few years ago, I watched a mother pushing her grocery cart as her two-year-old son walked beside her. Suddenly the little boy slipped and fell, but the mother didn't see him underneath her cart. As she pushed the card forward, the wheels rolled directly over her child's fingers. He instantly started shaking his reddened hand and screaming in pain.

What happened next still makes me shudder. The mother grabbed her little boy by the shoulder and jerked him behind her, yelling, "You stop crying this instant! That doesn't hurt and you know it!"

Any time you were told to stop feeling, you had to figure out what to do with your emotions. Maybe you learned how to talk yourself out of your feelings. Eventually, you may have translated the message "don't express" into "don't feel." Now, you just ignore your emotions or tell yourself they don't matter. But where did all those feelings go? For many people, these stifled feelings provide fuel for the battles of emotional eating.

CHANGING THE FAMILY RULES

The rules you learned in your family tend to stick with you and influence how you handle emotions as an adult. You might find it helpful to make a list of your family rules about emotions. Then consider how much these early messages affect the way you express your feelings now.

Do you still follow your old family rules or have you left them behind and adopted new methods for expressing how you feel? If you constantly got negative feedback about your feelings, you may hesitate to acknowledge or express them now. Don't let old rules keep you from becoming emotionally healthy. Except in rare cases of emotional abuse, most people can learn to overcome their family's influence on expressing emotions.

Sometimes, you can even go back and alter the rules you learned from your family. In our home, my parents kept the rules they'd each learned from their staunch German families. If you got mad, you could cry or yell (quietly) but you couldn't throw things or hit anyone. People weren't supposed to hug or kiss in public. "I love you" was reserved only for your spouse, not for your children.

After years of observing that my family rarely showed emotions, I decided to become more open in demonstrating love and affection. So in my twenties, I made a plan for how I would show love to my parents by giving them hugs and saying the words, "I love you." I knew my conservative parents might be uncomfortable with this, so I decided to gradually "teach" them how to show affection. My mother accepted my hugs quite readily, but getting a response from my father was a different story.

On one of my trips home, I carefully planned my strategy. When it was time for me to leave, I waited until my father was standing beside my car. Then I reached up, put my arms around him in a cautious hug and said, "I love you, Daddy." He just stood there like a huge brick, with his hands firmly at his sides. Then he muttered, "Yeah, well, okay then. Have a safe trip."

On my next visit, I did this again, giving him a gentle hug when I left. This time, he reached up and patted my arm. He was still quite embarrassed, but he didn't move away. From then on, each time I went home, I'd give him a hug and say "I love you," even though he always acted stiff and uneasy.

As time went on, though, my father grew more comfortable with my affection. Eventually, he started reaching up and patting my shoulders when I hugged him. One day, almost two years after I'd started this little project, my father surprised me by gruffly saying, "I love you, too." I was so moved by his unexpected response that I cried as I drove away.

My father slowly adapted to these changes in our family rules. In later years before his death, he hugged us kids easily and, in telephone conversations, he made of point of saying, "You know I love you."

Changing the way you show feelings doesn't have to be traumatic. You can start gradually, as I did, by expressing your emotions on a limited basis. Work at building a comfort level within yourself as well as with the people around you. Eventually, demonstrating your emotions will become alot easier.

Encouraging Your Emotions

Emotions are normal. You don't ask for them or have much say over them; they simply arrive. If most of your feelings are happy ones, you probably don't mind. But you may have trained yourself to run anytime you face uncomfortable emotions like anger or sadness.

Looking at your feelings isn't always enjoyable. Emotions make you face the truth about life. Sometimes they force you to consider decisions or changes you may not be ready for. If your feelings make you too uncomfortable, you may try to escape them entirely.

But blocking your emotions also means you have to avoid certain thoughts. So you continue to ignore your disappointment with your marriage or your children. You pretend you enjoy working at a meaningless job that never challenges you. You push aside long-standing bitterness over your childhood or your current life path.

Difficult emotions like anger and grief can make you feel like you're walking to the edge of a black hole. Because you can't see the bottom, you simply avoid looking into those dark feelings. Besides, if you start crying, you might not be able to stop. If you take the lid off your bitterness, you might just explode and say mean, hurtful things. So you keep the door to your bottled-up thoughts tightly closed.

Of course, to keep your feelings buried, you have to keep eating. So day after day, rather than give your emotions a chance to peek out, you use food to stuff them in. To get back in touch with your feelings, you may need to give up using food as a security blanket. At some point, you have to stop eating and look at what you've pushed below the surface.

Shirley tried to never think about her life. In reality, she felt insecure at her job, uneasy about her marriage, and afraid of the dark thoughts that made her feel so depressed. She said, "Food keeps me running from myself. As long as I keep eating, I don't have to face everything that's wrong in my life. So I just don't allow myself to stop."

WHERE DID YOUR EMOTIONS GO?

If you've stuffed your feelings for a long time, it may take some work to find them again. In all likelihood, your emotions aren't really gone, they've just become dormant. Reviving them might be as simple as adjusting the way you think about life.

All of your emotions live in the same part of your brain. You don't have separate compartments that allow you to lock up the uncomfortable ones while you have a party with the happy ones. This centralized storage area also controls the intensity of expressing your feelings.

When you were a child, you could scream your anger, sob your tears, and jump up and down when you felt happy. Little by little, you decreased the levels of how you showed your feelings. Instead of throwing a temper tantrum, you clenched your teeth or said a few bad words under your breath. When you were told to stop crying, you did, or at least you cried a lot more quietly.

From your parents, teachers, and even your friends, you learned how to be "proper" in showing your emotions. But some of what you learned may not have been accurate or even healthy. If you were taught to be selective in expressing your emotions, you may have chosen which feelings to keep and which ones to quietly push away.

As a result, perhaps you rarely show anger, and you certainly never cry. Instead of reacting when you feel sad or disappointed, you shove your thoughts aside and go on. In your mind, you believe you are in control of your feelings.

But emotions don't exist in isolation—they are all connected to each other. If you eliminate one category, you decrease the others as well. So if you choose to avoid anger, frustration, and sadness, you also diminish your ability to feel joy, love, and peacefulness.

THE EMOTIONAL BOX

If you block your emotions long enough, you can become so good at it that you stop feeling much of anything. You gradually build an invisible wall, sort of an "emotional box" around yourself to keep your feelings inside at all times. In this protected box, you continue to function as you always have. You go to work, you raise your children, you visit your mother. To the world, you look fine, but in truth, you've buried your authentic self.

Although the box helps you ignore uncomfortable emotions, it also numbs your positive feelings of love or happiness. Inside the box, you live in a neutral zone that makes you emotionally dull. Without the ability to feel and express emotions, you disconnect yourself from life. Eventually, your zest for living slips away and intimate relationships become a chore.

Perhaps you prefer keeping your emotions quiet. If you seem to be getting along fine without them, why bother uncovering your feelings? After all, you know your emotions can be very painful, and you'd rather not go through all that discomfort. Maybe,

The "Emotional Box"

Uncomfortable Emotions	Positive Emotions

Anger, Sadness, Loneliness, Boredom	Love, Happiness, Sexuality, Peace

in the past, talking about your feelings made things worse. Since it won't change anything, you may believe that it's futile to drag out your emotions.

Unfortunately, living in the emotional box isn't so great either. To keep your feelings from creeping in, you have to constantly insulate the walls, usually by stuffing yourself with food. At the same time, you may be afraid to crawl out of the box because if you do, you'll have start feeling things again, which doesn't appeal to you either.

Facing your emotions doesn't have to destroy you. When you take your feelings out of the dark and expose them, they're less scary, less threatening. You may discover that your grief, anger, and even bitterness aren't as intense as you remembered.

Once you bring your emotions out into the open, you may even feel relieved. You'll get a fresh view of how they connect to your eating. Knowing exactly which ones are driving you toward food can boost your confidence in coping with your feelings.

More than Mad, Glad, and Sad: Identifying Your Emotions

When you don't pay much attention to your feelings, it's easy to forget how to describe your emotions. Maybe you can think of only a few words, like angry, depressed, or happy. But within each of these categories lies an enormous range of descriptive words that can capture your feelings more accurately. Being precise makes identifying your emotions even more powerful.

Lots of emotions carry a range of intensity, from mild feelings like *upset* to major responses like *horrified*. Compare *explosive, furious,* or *anguished* to the less intense *irritated* or *frustrated*.

(continued on page 85)

Pressure Emotions

Intense pressure

Angry	Irate	Pissed off
Desperate	Irritated	Shocked
Explosive	Livid	Violated
Furious	Mad	
Horrified	Outraged	

Long-term anger

Aggravated	Exasperated	Offended
Annoyed	Frustrated	Smothered
Disgusted	Impatient	Ticked
Distressed	Irritated	Upset
Disturbed	Negative	

Stress

Belittled	Regretful	Revengeful
Bitter	Resentful	Shattered

Grouchiness

Consumed	Humiliated	Rushed
Cornered	Jealous	Stressed
Embarrassed	Overwhelmed	Tense
Flooded	Panicked	Threatened
Hassled	Pressed	Trapped
Hot	Pressured	

Irritation

Bitchy	Grouchy	Moody
Cranky	Grumpy	
Edgy	Irritable	

Empty Emotions

Emptiness

Alienated	Flat	Stifled
Apathetic	Hollow	Suffocated
Bored	Hopeless	Tired
Deprived	Insignificant	Unfulfilled
Disconnected	Passive	Weak
Distant	Sluggish	
Empty	Stale	

Sadness

Anguished	Drained	Numb
Betrayed	Griefstricken	Pessimistic
Blue	Helpless	Powerless
Dead	Hurt	Tearful
Depressed	Low	Unhappy
Discouraged	Miserable	Washed out
Down	Morose	

Fear

Afraid	Frightened	Torn
Anxious	Hesitant	Uncertain
Apprehensive	Insecure	Uncomfortable
Confused	Nervous	Unsure
Fearful	Scared	Worried

Loneliness

Abandoned	Isolated	Lost
Alone	Left out	Rejected
Burdened	Lonely	

Regret

Regretful	Shamed	Used
Remorseful	Sorry	

Positive Emotions

Happiness

Alive	Ecstatic	Happy
Anticipating	Elated	Inspired
Bouncy	Enthusiastic	Joyful
Bubbly	Euphoric	Lively
Charged	Excited	Overjoyed
Crazy	Exhilarated	Sparkly
Delighted	Exuberant	Tickled

Calm

Comfortable	Pleased	Serene
Content	Quiet	Successful
Grateful	Refreshed	Warm
Hopeful	Relaxed	Whole
Kindly	Relieved	Wonderful
Patient	Satisfied	
Peaceful	Secure	

Power

Adventuresome	Energetic	Stimulated
Amazed	Energized	Strong
Competent	Positive	Validated
Confident	Proud	Visionary
Empowered	Smart	Wise

Love

Adored	Cherished	Pretty
Affectionate	Fulfilled	Radiant
Appreciated	Glowing	Safe
Appreciative	Loved	Sexy
Attractive	Loving	Thrilled
Beautiful	Passionate	Turned on

Some feeling words don't prompt a tangible sensation but rather describe what you "think." For example, if you are debating between two job options, you may feel torn, confused, or hesitant. While these words don't necessarily evoke a physical response, they certainly provide an accurate description of what you're feeling.

To help you widen your range of emotions, study the list on pages 82–84. Go through each category a couple of times, particularly noticing words you haven't used in a while. After you read through these lists of emotions, see if you can think of any additional words that might accurately reflect how you feel.

"I FEEL . . . BECAUSE . . ."

Now it's time to identify your feelings in some real-life settings. Think of a recent situation that prompted an emotional response. Perhaps you wish you had handled something better in the past. Maybe you are facing an event or discussion you aren't looking forward to.

As you do this next exercise, keep the list of emotions in front of you, referring to it often to help you label your feelings accu-

---

"I feel . . . because . . . ."

On a blank piece of paper, draw a line down the middle from the top to the bottom. On the left side, write "I feel . . ."; on the right side, write "because." In the left column, begin writing words that describe your feelings about a situation, person, or event. Under the heading "because," add a reason or an explanation for why you feel this way. Use whatever words come to mind to describe your emotions and the reasons behind them. You can repeat words like "angry" as often as you like, just add a different explanation each time.

Keep your list simple, using one or two words to identify each feeling and a short phrase to describe why you feel that way. You can identify just a couple of feelings or fill an entire page with your emotions. Once you finish, read over your list and make sure you've accurately and completely addressed the situation.

---

rately. Since emotions vary so widely in intensity, be as specific as you can about what you feel. As you dig deeper, you may uncover many emotions besides the ones that initially show up.

For example, if you're feeling angry, decide whether you're actually *livid, bitter,* or *overwhelmed*. Maybe your feelings are less intense, and you're just *annoyed, irritated,* or *grouchy*. Suppose you're depressed over a relationship breakup. In addition to feeling *down, tearful,* or *sad,* look for other words that fit. Maybe you also feel *lonely, discouraged, disappointed,* or *abandoned*.

Identifying your emotions brings them out into the open. And once you see the whole picture, you aren't as likely to reach for food to cover up what you feel. You don't even have to write the words down to be able to identify your feelings. You can just think them or even say them to your steering wheel as you drive.

The "I feel... because..." exercise can help you explore your feelings in a wide range of life circumstances—from general thoughts about your job or your home to specific situations like a fight with your spouse.

You might start by taking a mental sweep of your present situation and describing your thoughts about life in general. Consider *all* the areas that currently affect you, including both positive, happy ones and difficult or challenging ones. Here's an example.

I feel...	because...
Happy	my three children are wonderful.
Frustrated	I can't seem to get caught up.
Stressed	I'm under a lot of pressure at work.
Worried	my company is considering layoffs.
Thrilled	I love my new house.
Content	I have a great husband.

The lost promotion. Over the past year, Cheryl had worked hard at her job, putting in lots of overtime and skipping lunches to meet deadlines and finish reports. When a promotion opportunity came up, she felt confident she would get it. Unexpectedly, Cheryl's boss announced that the position had been given to Karen, another employee, who hadn't put in the extensive work that Cheryl had. After months of working toward this promotion, Cheryl was furious that she wasn't rewarded or appreciated for her efforts. Normally, this would have sent her toward an eating binge of fast foods and cheesecake. But this time, she sat down and wrote a list of her emotions, using "I feel . . . because. . . ."

I feel . . .	because . . .
Outraged	Karen got the promotion, not me.
Resentful	she's so manipulative.
Humiliated	friends were sure I'd get it.
Trapped	job feels dead-end now.
Furious	I worked so hard for nothing.
Disgusted	boss plays favorites.
Worn out	I'm fighting to get ahead.
Bitter	life isn't fair.
Angry and resentful	my boss never shows appreciation.

Completing her list helped Cheryl recognize that her feelings were appropriate considering the situation. So she decided to look for ways to deal with her anger and frustration. First, she went to her exercise class and worked off some of her tension. Later that evening, she called a friend and brainstormed ways she could handle her current job while exploring other work options. Then she took a relaxing bath and went to bed, exhausted but proud of the fact she hadn't slipped into her old pattern of eating to cope with her anger.

When you successfully identify your feelings, you find the power to change your response. Giving in to a double cheeseburger might have made Cheryl feel better for the moment, but it wouldn't have solved the problem. By postponing the temptation to shove her anger down with food, she was able to process her feelings and recognize better ways to handle them.

Sometimes your original response will shift as you write down your feelings. When you face a situation that makes you want to send out for pizza or shove a bag of chips into your mouth, postpone eating until you've figured out exactly what you're feeling. Use the "I feel . . . because . . ." exercise to dilute the intensity of your emotions and give yourself time to come up with a better solution.

When feelings elude you. What if you can't figure out what you're feeling? Sometimes you won't be able to come up with words that match your emotions about a particular situation. In this case, ask yourself this: "If I knew what I was feeling, what would it be?" This simple question can take you past your mental roadblocks and help you find words that fit. Go back to the list of emotions and search again for an accurate description of what you're feeling at the moment.

Be careful not to talk yourself out of your emotions. Any time you say, "I shouldn't be so upset," you're trying to ignore or suppress what you actually feel. If you go through a difficult or uncomfortable experience, you're entitled to feel "so upset." It's what you do with your upset that determines whether or not you stuff it down with food.

WHERE DOES GUILT FIT?

Despite our common use of the word, guilt is not really an emotion. When you say you "feel guilty" about a behavior, you're not describing a feeling. Instead, the word "guilty" serves as a cover-up for a variety of less acceptable emotions. Any time you feel guilty about something, ask yourself the following question: *"If I wasn't feeling guilty, what would I be feeling?"*

When you peek underneath guilty feelings, you discover a whole range of emotions. Suppose you ate a piece of cake that wasn't on your diet plan. To get beyond "feeling guilty," consider what else is going on. Maybe you feel *disappointed* because you couldn't resist a temptation or *frustrated* because you fell off your diet. Perhaps you're afraid you'll never lose weight or that your spouse will yell at you.

Saying you feel guilty about eating cake is often easier than facing the truth. When you identify your *real* feelings, however, you discover the insecurity and disappointment that prompted you to eat the cake. You might not have recognized these feelings if you hadn't looked beyond feeling guilty.

Cassie's aging parents lived several hundred miles away from her. She knew she should see them more often, but every time she returned home after visiting them, she went into an eating frenzy. She assumed her food struggles were related to "feeling guilty" about not visiting them sooner or doing more things for them.

When she made a list of what she felt outside of "guilty," Cassie began to understand why she disliked going home.

I feel...	because...
Angry	they expect me to visit a lot.
Frustrated	lack of money keeps me from flying home often.
Afraid	they'll think I've abandoned them.
Devastated	they're going downhill so fast.
Worried	they might need nursing home care soon.
Irritated	they don't act like they appreciate me.
Bitter	they've ignored me for much of my life.
Resentful	my brother doesn't take his turn at visiting.

Cassie realized she had many conflicting emotions about her parents and their current situation. Instead of covering her thoughts by feeling guilty, she processed what she *really* felt. Once she understood her emotions and shifted her attitude, Cassie was able to stop her eating binges.

Saying you feel guilty might seem like an easy way out. But digging underneath those words helps you face emotions you were trying to avoid. By uncovering your hidden feelings, you can create solutions for taking care of them instead of eating them away.

Reviving Lost Feelings

If you've lost touch with your emotions, you may need to pull some of them back up to a conscious level. Recovering your feelings doesn't mean you have to start pounding your fists and screaming out your anger, although you may eventually reach that point. You simply need to move out of the neutral zone and rebuild your enthusiasm for life.

To bring your emotions back up to the surface, you first have to provoke your feelings, then allow yourself to experience them. One way to revive feelings is to rent movies that you know will prompt an emotional response. Watch a tragically sad movie, then go ahead and cry. Invite a group of friends over to a comedy night, then pull out movies that make you laugh until your stomachs hurt.

If you've forgotten how anger feels, go to an animal shelter that houses abused pets. Stand in front of their cages and try to imagine the pain they've endured. Allow the intensity of your feelings to build as you picture the cruelty experienced by these animals. Don't just feel sad for them—feel *angry*! Let that emotion surface in other areas of your life instead of using food to keep it buried.

THE COURAGE TO FEEL

Attaching words to your emotions puts you in a stronger position to deal with them. But feeling your emotions also takes courage. Once you recognize an emotion, allow yourself to sit with it. Hold it, look at it, then describe it by adding more words. For example, if you feel angry or sad, dissect these emotions into tinier pieces and search for accurate words to explain them. Use the emotions list shown earlier in this chapter for help in labeling your feelings.

As you explore ways to stop the patterns of emotional eating, you won't always like the solution. You may unearth pain you buried long ago, hoping never to face it again. And food will always lure you with the promise of an easy escape.

But never give up on your efforts. Facing your emotions will give you an amazing edge in adhering to your weight-management goals. When you no longer require food to appease your emotions, it will be much easier to stay on your diet and exercise program.

CHAPTER SIX

Expressing, Not Stuffing

AFTER TWENTY-SEVEN YEARS of marriage, Lucy had hoped her life would be more enjoyable. Instead, she felt angry and bitter toward her husband, Mark, and how he ignored her. Between the hours he spent working, visiting his elderly mother, and playing poker with his buddies, Mark was away most of the time. In her efforts to escape her loneliness and resentment, Lucy ate. For many years, food was her only source of relief and comfort.

When she joined a new weight-loss program, Lucy participated in a journal-writing group that explored emotional issues. One afternoon, after an angry telephone conversation with Mark, she grabbed a can of potato chips, then took out her notebook and began to write.

Inside I feel a slow burn. I desperately try to suppress the anger that's building to a rage in the pit of my stomach. My face feels red and hot. I hate anger! I've always hated it. I never want to feel it, so I'll do anything to avoid it. My anger feels like a raging bull facing the red canvas that taunts me toward destruction. It terrifies me, and I must make it go away.

I know! I'll open the fresh, round container of potato chips. Yes, that will do it. As I reach for the familiar red cylinder, my conscience warns, "I shouldn't be eating this."

But the force is too great and guilt lasts only momentarily. The top of the can pries off easily, and as quickly as my hand will move, I pull out a stack of curved golden morsels. One lifts instantly to my mouth where my teeth mash it with a vengeance. Before I realize it, I have devoured six or seven more.

The sound is soothing, like water lapping softly on the beach. Listening to the rhythm of the waves inside my head encourages me to keep eating. The lingering taste of salt, like the salt of the sea, rocks me into calmness and the raging anger begins to slip away.

Gently, even the reason for the anger washes out to sea. As I continue to chew, it floats so far away that even straining can't bring it back. The bullfighter has slain his victim. Now the red canvas with its teasing bright color may be folded and stowed away. The sea is calm, and I may rest. —Lucy

When she read her journal entry, Lucy was amazed at the power and intensity of her anger. She also recognized that, for years, she had been stuffing her anger away with food. As Lucy uncovered her feelings of resentment and bitterness toward Mark—and even their children—she decided it was time to cope with her feelings instead of eating them away. After another argument with Mark a few days later, here's how she recorded her thoughts.

Today I must look at my anger. What caused it? Will it hurt me? Life is not what I pictured it would be and my anger may be related to that as much as the moment. But can I face it? Like a pressure cooker steaming on the burner far too long, I fear I will burst, sending remnants of past issues stuffed within me too long in every direction. Shall I reach for the red cylinder and push the anger deep down to calm the sea? I think not. Today I will meet the issue straight on. The bullfighter will not win. The red canvas will remain in the cupboard and I will face my anger instead of reaching to food for relief. —Lucy

The Power of Expressing Emotions

Grief, anger, disappointment, bitterness, resentment—all of these cause emotional pain. When you can't deal with these feelings, it's easy to let food become the drug that soothes them away. But emotional eating just creates another layer of pain. The only way to escape the trap of eating instead of feeling is to learn other ways to manage your emotions.

In this chapter, you'll learn how to build powerful skills that will make you stronger and more comfortable with all levels of emotional coping. Along with learning how to talk about your feelings more easily, you'll also discover how to express them through music, journal writing, and physical touch.

Expressing your emotions without food won't always be easy. You might stumble a lot during your early attempts to face and express your feelings. But don't give up just because something doesn't work the first time. Fine-tune your skills, then try again. With practice, you'll eventually get better at discussing your emotions and managing them in healthier ways.

What Gets in Your Way?

Have you ever tried to talk about your feelings, but then had the entire discussion blow up in your face? Or has telling someone how you felt ever made the situation worse? If things have gone badly when you've expressed your emotions, you might be afraid to say something the next time.

So where do you start? If you haven't talked about your feelings for a long time, pulling them out into the open will take some effort. First, it helps if you recognize some of the barriers that prevent you from expressing how you feel. Second, you need to develop an effective set of tools that will ensure you get the results you want.

If you can't bring yourself to talk about your emotions, you need to figure out what gets in the way of discussing them. Then you have to figure out how to work around these barriers and express your feelings *anyway*.

FEAR OF REJECTION

"If I tell you how I feel, you'll get mad."

Does this sound familiar? If you worry about how people will react when you express your emotions, you may decide it's easier to keep your thoughts to yourself. Speaking up takes courage, especially when you think your feelings might be rejected.

See if any of these fears or concerns keep you from talking about your emotions.

• I'll say it "wrong" or my words will sound dumb.
• I could jeopardize my relationship or harm my chance of a promotion at work.
• People will get upset about how I feel.
• I need to protect others from feeling hurt.
• I could be at risk for retribution or even physical abuse.
• In this situation, I don't feel safe enough to discuss my feelings.
• I might be rejected or abandoned.

Even though it's difficult, you need to overcome your fear of people's reactions. Work on building your self-esteem and your confidence so you feel stronger about speaking up. You might also focus on communication skills so you can be assertive rather than aggressive in your conversations.

"I Shouldn't Feel This Way"

Do you ever talk yourself out of having a feeling because you don't think it's appropriate? Maybe you worry that you're "too sensitive" or that your feelings are "wrong." If you don't trust your own reaction to intense emotions like anger or hurt, you might decide to avoid feeling them.

Whenever you tell yourself "I shouldn't feel this way," you essentially pretend you aren't having an emotion. But like Lucy and her resentment, ignoring what you feel won't make it go away. Emotions have to go somewhere. Without a way to let your feelings out, you'll probably keep reaching for food to push them away.

"You Shouldn't Feel This Way"

Sometimes, other people will try to keep you from expressing your feelings because it makes them uncomfortable. You may hear things like "You shouldn't feel that way" or "You're overreacting" or "You're wrong."

Telling someone how to feel is a method of control. These people may want you to just give in and say what *they* want to hear instead of what you really feel. Or they may not want you to have a feeling at all.

Brian hated to see his wife cry. So whenever she got tearful about something, he would beg her to stop.

I couldn't stand to be around tears. They made me feel helpless and unsure of myself. Because her crying made me so uncomfortable, I never allowed her to be sad. Finally I realized that when I told her to stop crying, I actually wanted her to stop feeling. —Brian

In my work as a nurse, I often watched people avoid discussing a family member's life-threatening illness. They would say things like "We don't think our mother will be able to handle it, so we won't tell her what the doctor said." What they really mean is "We can't handle how we will feel if we have to watch her reaction."

Usually, the mother already suspected the seriousness of her diagnosis. But since her family members couldn't deal with their own pain, she had no chance to talk about her own feelings. Being healthy in your own emotions requires that you also let others experience and express what they feel.

ATTACKING OR BLAMING

If you start a conversation by saying "You make me so mad" or "It's your fault I feel this way," you won't get far in resolving your emotions. Instead of reflecting how you feel, these statements lash out at the other person. They also make people defensive and likely to resist your comments. In a heated discussion, you may end up taking turns blaming or criticizing each other rather than sharing your feelings.

Be careful about using your emotions to manipulate people or get revenge. Attacking someone else doesn't bring you healing. It only harms relationships and breeds more negative feelings. If your goal is to get even, punish, or teach a lesson, you aren't expressing your emotions in a healthy way.

Do you ever save up your feelings, then suddenly blast them everywhere? If you keep silent for too long, your emotions can build to such a pressure point that when you finally express them, it's easy to explode and dump the whole truck. If you're bottling up your feelings and can't seem to talk about them, explore them in other ways. Consider describing them in a journal or talking to a counselor, who can encourage you to get your feelings out instead of letting them blow up.

When you're ready to talk about your feelings, make sure you have a receptive audience. If there's a possibility of abuse or retaliation, you may need to find a different avenue for working through your emotions. In the same way, if you are around someone who is drunk or high, it's best to postpone discussing your emotions until later. If your emotional struggle involves an authoritarian boss or a demanding parent, you may need to look for another option. In these cases, it might be best to not tell your feelings to the person involved and talk to someone else instead.

FATIGUE, ILLNESS, OR STRESS

Be careful about expressing your feelings when you're tired or overwhelmed. As fatigue and stress levels climb, your ability to communicate effectively drops. The same thing is true when you're recovering from an injury or an illness.

When you're physically worn out, it's hard to sort out your feelings and express them kindly. Think about how you feel after you've spent several days traveling or caring for a sick child or parent. In fact, anything that challenges your patience will also compromise your ability to tactfully discuss how you feel.

Monitor how you handle things such as stress or fatigue. Sometimes a physical need can appear to be an emotional one. After a long, hard day, take time to rest and regroup before you launch into a conversation about emotions. Learn to ask "Am I angry or am I exhausted?" Then decide whether it's critical that you talk immediately or if you should just get some sleep.

What Makes It Work?

You don't have to express your emotions perfectly to prevent yourself from reaching for food, you just need to keep working at it. But you can make the process easier by planning a few things ahead of time.

A SAFE ENVIRONMENT

Sharing your deeper thoughts and feelings takes being in a situation where you feel emotionally safe. Choose your audience carefully. When you get ready to discuss your emotions, you want to know you'll be "heard" and that what you feel will be respected and valued, not scoffed at or belittled.

Sometimes it makes sense to speak directly to the one who prompted your feelings. But other times you may be better off talking to someone else such as a trusted friend or colleague. If you are working through a particularly difficult issue, consider discussing your feelings with a therapist, a minister, or a life coach.

Sometimes, you can be your own best audience, working out your feelings through self-talk, writing, exercise, and other expressive activities. You can even stay at home some evening and describe your emotions to your pet. Just do something that gets the words out instead of holding them inside.

WHAT'S THE REAL NEED?

Your emotions can get tangled up with a lot of other issues. Look at your life and decide whether you're facing a bigger problem than just expressing what you feel. Are you struggling with an impossible job situation or a relationship that's on the rocks? If so, consider whether you need to set healthier boundaries and stop letting yourself be manipulated.

Fixing a broken relationship takes more than expressing emotions. Although talking about your feelings is important, you may also need to spend more time together or improve how you communicate. If you seem to be eating because of a relationship struggle, divide the situation into smaller parts. Are you upset because your partner always yells at you during arguments? Or is the problem related to not having enough time together? Decide what you can do to improve specific areas, such as how you speak to one another on the phone.

Suppose you always binge after spending a weekend with your fiancé. Instead of eating your feelings every Sunday night, stop to figure out what's going on. What's missing in the relationship? What do you need right now that you aren't getting? Maybe you know intuitively that it's time to break up, but you can't quite bring yourself to do it.

The longer you postpone making changes, the more you'll keep reaching for food. Start working through your emotions by using the exercise "I feel...because..." or by asking "What do I need?" Then talk to another person about your difficulty with coping. As you uncover your feelings and express them, you'll eventually get to the heart of your emotional eating.

WHOSE PROBLEM IS IT?

Do you try to "fix" other people's feelings? If you get upset at how someone else handles emotions, ask yourself "Whose problem is it and do I want to make it mine?" Look beyond the feelings themselves to see if you're dealing with a relationship issue, a communication problem, or an actual need to express a feeling.

Instead of trying to control other people's emotions, allow them to feel whatever they want. I used to complain a lot about my husband's anger over his job. One day he glared at me and said, "This is my problem, and if I want to be mad about it, let me be mad."

BE KIND

If you've repressed your feelings for a long time, you may need to start small instead of letting go with both barrels. Expressing your emotions doesn't give you license to be mean or cause harm. If necessary, practice ahead of time so you can talk about your feelings in a kind, gentle manner. Instead of intending to hurt someone, begin with a sincere desire to communicate.

If the person you're talking to becomes defensive or starts throwing angry words at you, slow down and listen to what's being said. Instead of interrupting or getting upset, allow the other person to talk for a while. Then formulate new "I feel" statements and ask for permission to share your additional thoughts.

Uncovering the Layers

Expressing a feeling doesn't always bring instant relief. Deeper emotions often have many layers that need to be worked through one at a time. Sometimes you'll express something, feel better, then have the emotions return.

If your feelings are still there, don't assume you didn't do it right. Just express them again and peel off another layer. Some intense feelings such as grief will never go away completely, but expressing them weakens their intensity and moves you closer to healing.

Letting Go of Emotions

When you identify an emotion, consider how much meaning you attach to that particular feeling. Is it important? If you ignore it, will it affect you in some negative way? Or are you dealing with a "file and forget" issue? If you get stuck on every small irritation, you can waste a lot of time working on trivial emotions.

Whenever you get angry at drivers, sales clerks, or telephone solicitors, sort through what you feel. Do you really need to stew over these irritations and stomp around in frustration? Or could you say to yourself "that made me mad," then simply get over it?

Question whether a minor issue is worth an angry interaction. When you get into an emotionally charged situation, think about whether it will be important an hour from now. Like fishing in a stocked pond, be willing to let the "little ones" go.

Relax the Feelings

Often you can decrease the intensity of difficult emotions by processing them and thinking them through. In some cases, you can sidestep an emotional response just by calming yourself down and sorting out the situation. You might change your expectations about how others "should" react.

Sometimes all you need is to relax or get some rest. Deep breathing, imagery, or meditation often defuse intense feelings like bitterness or resentment. Let go of tension or anger by taking a warm bath or sitting quietly, surrounded by candles. Just be sure you're truly getting resolution, not just pushing your feelings away.

Draw on Music

Have you ever noticed how listening to music changes your mood or calms your emotions? You can actually alter your physical responses by varying the type of music you choose. As your body absorbs the beat and vibrations from a song, it adapts your heart rate, blood pressure, and breathing to mimic the rhythm of the music.

If you're tired, depressed, or lonely, don't pull out your romantic ballads or slow country songs. To change your mood, choose bright, forceful songs, especially ones with a fast, upbeat tempo. When you want to brighten a down mood, play music that has a beat faster than your heart rate. To determine the beat of a song, tap your foot or a pencil in rhythm to the music, then count the number of taps per minute. A musical rhythm that exceeds 70 or 80 beats a minute will usually do the job.

In the same way, when you need to calm down or soothe away anger or other intense emotions, select music with a gentle rhythmic sound. Look for "new age" instrumental recordings, classical works, or any quiet, relaxing music. As you listen to the songs, focus on breathing more slowly and deeply, allowing the music to lull you into a calmer state of mind.

Let Yourself Cry

Tears are important. If you resist the urge to cry, you lose an important outlet for expressing sadness or hurt as well as anger. Don't allow the need to "be strong" keep you from crying. Even though you may hate tears, sobbing your heart out can be therapeutic and healing. So when tears start welling up, let them do their work, releasing emotions that otherwise might be stuffed deep inside.

For many years, I avoided crying because it messed up my contacts and gave me a headache. But when I began seeing a therapist about my grief issues, I realized I was eating instead of crying. So I made the decision to allow crying back into my life as a way to express my feelings. Now when my tears come, I celebrate because they show my emotions are alive, not pushed into an emotional box.

When You Can't Let Go

If you can't seem to let go of a feeling, look at why you want to hold on to it so badly. What are you getting out of it? Consider what keeps you attached to long-standing feelings like anger or bitterness. What are you afraid will happen if you give up those feelings?

Fear of Change

Perhaps letting go of your anger means you'd have to allow more intimacy or be more accepting of a situation. With relationship issues, you might lose your ability to punish the other person. So look carefully at areas you don't really want to change. If getting a new job or leaving a relationship feels too scary, you may be using your emotions to protect yourself from taking a step you aren't ready for.

Do you hold on to your emotions because you don't want to lose your excuse for overeating? If you aren't ready to live without food as a source of emotional comfort, you may not want to get past your bad feelings.

After three years of marriage, Ron's wife had an affair, then eventually left him for the other man. A short time later, she married her new boyfriend, and they seemed quite happy in their new life.

When Ron came to my weight-loss clinic, he talked at length about his intense sadness and depression over the loss of the relationship. "Lots of days, I still cry because I miss her so much. I know I'm eating all the time to fill the void, but I just can't seem to get over it."

When I asked Ron how long it had been since the relationship ended, he answered, "Nine years!" To me, Ron didn't sound like he wanted to get over it. Besides, his ongoing grief provided an excuse for his troubled eating. Ron's participation in the weight-loss program was short-lived because at that moment, he didn't want to let go of his grief.

A MATTER OF PRINCIPLE

Although they weren't close friends, Kevin and his neighbor usually got along just fine. But one day, the neighbor borrowed Kevin's lawnmower and when he returned it, the blade was broken. Initially, Kevin tried to be nice, asking his neighbor if he knew what had caused the blade to snap and if he'd be willing to pay for a new one.

The neighbor became quite defensive, saying the blade must have been worn out and that it wasn't his fault. The discussion escalated until they both got angry. Finally, Kevin decided he'd had enough and he stomped into his house.

But for years, whenever he thought about that day, Kevin felt angry all over again. He refused to speak to his neighbor and smooth things out. Because the situation was a matter of "principle," he believed his feelings were legitimate.

Be careful with holding on to your feelings for the sake of "principle." Often the stance you defend so intensely isn't a big deal in the long run. I'm not suggesting you compromise your values of honesty and integrity. But, don't get sucked into a battle of emotions over something that won't matter at all in a few months or a year.

The same is true with demanding an apology. If you refuse to forgive someone until you get an apology, you risk storing your anger for a long time. Usually, the other person goes on with life while you stew with your anger, stuffing food to cope with something you think will hurt them. The person on the receiving end of this one-sided agreement may not even know it's a problem, yet you pay a high price for holding on to your feelings.

REHASHING A FEELING

Do you ever find yourself complaining about the same problem over and over? As you describe how upset you are, you get upset all over again. If it seems like you're whining or complaining, you probably are. Rehashing or repeating the same stories doesn't bring resolution and healing, it just keeps the pain active.

To determine whether you're just rehashing your feelings, go back to your motives. Are you trying to get revenge or control a relationship? Or are you looking deep inside and expressing your true feelings as a way to bring healing?

LET THEM GO

Here's a technique to help you identify feelings, then let them go. When a driver cuts you off in traffic or someone is rude to you at a store, allow your anger or irritation to move through your brain. Look closely at the feelings, make sure they are accurate, then say to yourself, "I got it!"

Then visualize those emotions flowing down your arms and on out through your fingertips. You might even stretch your arm out toward the offending car or person to symbolize you have completed your work and that you're letting the feelings go.

A counselor once told me, "Go ahead and feel it; just don't feel it all day." If you tend to hold on to "small-time emotions," practice setting a time limit on them. To do this, write your feelings on a piece of paper or mentally list your emotions about a situation. Then decide how long you want to hold on to the feelings—from a few minutes to several hours.

Either place the paper or mentally tuck your thoughts into the palm of your hand. Close your fist tightly around the feelings. At the end of your designated time limit, open your hand and throw the paper away or mentally send the thoughts into outer space.

When you deal with an uncomfortable emotion, work hard to allow it, express it, and let it go. Once you release a feeling, be sure to completely let go of it. Don't pick it up again or allow it to creep back into your thoughts. If you can't seem to get rid of a bad feeling, repeat the process of setting a time limit. Once again, decide how long to hold on to your emotion, then when the time is up, let it go.

How to Talk about Feelings

To get your feelings out, you have to start talking about them. No more bottling them up, then eating to keep them stuffed inside. But how do you begin? Here are a few ideas that can make the process go a lot easier.

HAVE A WARM-UP

Before you start discussing your feelings, pave the way by planning for the conversation. Consider whether the timing and the environment are appropriate. When people are rushing off to a meeting or to baseball practice, they may not have the patience to listen to you. If your mother-in-law is eavesdropping on the conversation, your spouse might not be very receptive to your discussion.

Be sensitive to energy levels, both yours and the other person's. If people are exhausted or hungry after a long workday, wait until they've rested and eaten a meal before you begin describing your emotions.

Learn how to set the stage. To discuss emotions, you first have to get the other person's attention, then say things in ways that don't start a fire. If your discussions don't go well in the beginning, feel free to tell others, "I'm learning how to express my feelings better. Please bear with me as I practice."

Pay attention to the way you're pointing when you express your emotions. Whenever possible, use "I" statements such as "I feel angry," not "You make me angry." Always focus on *your feelings*, not the other person or their actions. Think in terms of "I feel, I need, I want . . ." rather than attacking the other person with "You never, you should, you caused it."

If you use your emotions to attack or punish someone, you might feel smug when you're finished. But your feelings won't be resolved; in fact, they'll probably come back. And when they do, you may go back to emotional eating, since "expressing your feelings didn't work."

INVITE AND ARRANGE

Unless the situation is urgent, ask the other person, "Is this a good time to talk?" Right before your boss has to conduct a staff meeting might not be good timing for a discussion about emotions. And if your night-owl teen gets an energy boost around midnight, you might need to stay up late to have a meaningful chat.

Start your visit with a check-in on how the person is doing. Attempt to build a connection by asking about the day or some aspect of life. Be prepared to take risks. When you start sharing your feelings with other people, you can't always predict how they will respond.

HOW TO SAY IT

When you're ready to talk, feel free to draw from many different methods. You can start by asking someone to sit down and saying, "I need to talk to you." Another option is to write a list of "I feel . . . because . . ." statements, then read it to the person involved. Sometimes you just need a listening ear so you can get things off your chest. In that case, vent your emotions to a good friend or a fam-

---

"I feel, I want, I'll help"

Begin by telling someone what you feel, then follow up with a request that the behavior be altered or stopped. Finish by offering to help the other person make the changes. When you get angry or upset, this technique will help you express your feelings in a way that doesn't attack the other person or make them defensive. Here's the sequence of statements.

• When _____, I feel _____.

• Instead I want _____.

• How can I help you do this? _____.

---

ily member, or perhaps talk to your apartment walls or your steering wheel.

Sometimes it helps to have a structured technique to help you express yourself accurately. This next approach shows how to state your feelings and desires in a specific order that nearly always results in the changes you want.

To use this method effectively, always begin by identifying the situation that's bothering you. Start with the specific phrases, "When I see" or "When this happens," then add a description of the problem. Whenever possible, use an "I" statement or a factual observation. By depersonalizing your comments and leaving out any reference to the other person, you don't give them a reason to become defensive.

For example, instead of saying, "When *you leave* your dirty clothes on the floor" consider phrasing it as "When *I see* your dirty clothes on the floor." There is a subtle but powerful difference between these two statements. Instead of blaming or attacking, you allow the possibility that *anyone* could have put the clothes on the floor.

After you've identified the problem, say "I feel..." and fill in your emotions about the situation. Think about this ahead of time to be sure you describe your feelings accurately.

Next, tell the person what you want *in place of* the offending behavior. If at all possible, don't use the word "you." Instead, simply state the action you want. With the laundry problem, you might say, "Instead, I want the clothes put into the hamper or clothes basket."

Finally, add an invitation to help, such as "Would you like to have a laundry basket in your own closet? Can I do anything else to make this easier for you?" By asking people how you can help them comply with your request, you increase the likelihood of getting their cooperation.

Allison's husband had gotten into the habit of spending three or four nights a week playing golf or bowling with his friends. Although they actually had a good marriage, Allison eventually got tired of being home alone. She came up with the following terms to discuss her feelings with her husband.

When I'm home by myself several evenings a week, I feel lonely and sad. I want to have your company on more evenings. How could I help you get the relaxation you need from your work stress, yet not be away as much?
—Allison

While sometimes it's tricky to do this, remember to focus on yourself and your feelings, not on the other person. Notice when Allison described the situation, she did not say, "When you are gone several evenings..." Even though it's a subtle difference, your message will be heard a lot differently, and you're more likely to get a positive response to your request.

BE SPECIFIC

When you identify what you want, avoid using vague terms or words with a judgmental meaning such as responsible, mature, or nice. No one except you knows exactly what you mean by these words. While you may have a clear image of a "responsible" person, your employee may not hold the same definition. You'll get a much better response if you state precisely what you want, using words that are clear and specific.

When Valerie went back to school, her husband agreed to take care of their home one evening a week. He knew he was supposed to feed the kids and get them ready for bed. But week after week, he left the dirty dishes on the table and the children's clothes strewn all over the floor. Valerie constantly tried to change his behavior by saying she wanted him to be more responsible around the house.

I suspected her husband didn't know what she meant by the word "responsible." He assumed that by feeding the kids and spending the evening with them, he was doing his job well. When I showed Valerie the "I see" technique, she came up with a new sequence to express her feelings. Before she left for the next class meeting, she told her husband what she wanted.

When I come home after class and I see the dirty dishes on the table and the kids' clothes lying on the floor, I feel angry and frustrated. I want the dishes put into the dishwasher and their clothes laid in a pile on their dressers. Would you like help with any of that, such as loading the dishwasher? —Valerie

Valerie's husband acted surprised, but agreed to do what he could. The next time Valerie arrived home after her class, she found the house was spotless, and those things done exactly as she requested.

Other Ways to Express Emotions

Most of the time, people express their emotions by talking about them. But as long as you move toward resolution and healing, you can use any method that works. You may need to use a combination of several things, especially with difficult issues or intense emotional struggles.

Some of the following methods don't technically involve expressing emotions, yet they help you get your feelings out and deal with them. Remember, the goal is to *cope* with your feelings, not *eat them*.

FIND OTHER OUTLETS

When you need to process uncomfortable emotions, look for a way to release the feelings or decrease their power over you. Intense exercise or other physical activity like kickboxing or hitting a punching bag can relieve feelings of anger or frustration. A long walk or bike ride may help dissolve tension, stress, or even irritation.

Angela's work at a crisis counseling center often left her feeling troubled, tense, or upset at the end of the day. When she first started the job, she would go home after work and grab a big bag of potato chips or cookies to settle her mind down after the intensity of the day. Then she decided to try something new.

I made it a habit to stop at the recreation center on the way home and process my thoughts over a long walk. I told myself that I would walk until I felt better, which meant I'd stay until my tension and troubled thoughts from the day were gone. Usually I walked for twenty or thirty minutes, but occasionally it took an hour to reach the point of feeling better. —Angela

Physical activity also works great for sad or empty feelings like depression, loneliness, or grief. With these feelings, there's a tendency to sit down and sink lower into them. Getting active forces you to move around and get your blood flowing.

Hug Someone

Touch makes you real. It validates your existence and helps you believe you are valuable as a person. If your life is lacking in touch, you're missing out on a way to connect with a lot of your feelings.

Think about the power of a hug. With hugs, you can express a range of positive feelings including love, joy, appreciation, concern, and sympathy. Besides healing your heart, genuine hugs can build your confidence and self-esteem better than words. Hugs allow you to share yourself openly and show people how much you care about them.

Hugs need to be felt. People often give "air hugs"—when they just briefly touch or pat each other on the shoulder. Sometimes, that's all that's socially appropriate. But when it becomes the only way you touch other people, you miss out on an important way to express your feelings.

First-timer hug. If you're just getting started with hugging, practice with someone you feel comfortable with. Standing face to face, reach your arms up and around each other, then briefly squeeze each other's shoulders. Appreciate the warmth of touching someone's skin or pressing your arms against another person.

Notice whether you tend to pat or slap the other person's back at the end of your hug. Often people of the same sex, particularly males, will do this when they hug each other. Patting the other person neutralizes the sexuality of the hug, decreasing the potential of sexual thoughts related to touching someone.

Patting the other person is a common social style, but it changes the nature of a hug. Although giving a "patting hug" might feel safer, you sacrifice the benefit of enjoying a warm, connecting touch.

Heart-to-heart hug. Tell someone you want the two of you to feel the beat of each other's heart as part of a hug. Then position the left half of your body over the other person's left chest, aligning the general areas of your hearts. Wrap your arms tightly around each other and strain to feel a heartbeat. Although you might not actually feel each other's heartbeat, this exercise gives you a wonderful excuse for holding someone close.

Heart-to-heart hugs provide a great way to show love to anyone, but they work especially well with children. When you do a heart-to-heart hug with small children, kneel in front of them or have them stand on stairs so your shoulders are at about equal height. Because it feels like a game, most kids love the idea of hugging you to feel your heartbeat. In fact, if you can convince your teenagers to try this, you may get your first real hug from them in years.

Holding hug. Another great way to appreciate touch is to turn a hug into a "hold." Again, do this with someone you feel safe with, such as your life partner or a family member. Ask the other person to hug you for ten seconds while you both count the time off in your heads. Holding hugs are very healing. They can also help you feel reconnected with someone you want to be close to.

Finding people to hug. To get more touch into your life, search out people you can hug safely, then do it. Start letting your friends and relatives know you like to show your feelings by giving hugs. If necessary, teach people around you that hugs and touching are okay.

You might tell people you have to fulfill an assignment and ask them to help you practice your new types of hugs. Standing close to someone and soaking up the sense of touch for a few seconds can provide a great way to express a lot of your emotions.

If you don't have anyone available for safe hugging, look for places where touch will be valued and appreciated. Visit a nursing home or assisted-living center and ask about residents who rarely have visitors or whose families live far away. Spend some time getting acquainted, then when you leave, ask if you can give them a hug. Elderly people are often touch-deprived and they love to have someone reach out to them with a hug.

Whenever you wish to offer a hug to someone you don't know well, *always* ask permission ("May I give you a hug?"). People with a history of physical or sexual abuse may be anxious or very uncomfortable when they're hugged or touched. Be sensitive to their needs; don't just barge into their personal space.

WRITE YOUR FEELINGS DOWN

Getting words out of your head is a necessary part of expressing your emotions. But what if you don't have anyone to talk to? You can express your feelings in many ways that don't involve saying the words out loud.

Journal writing. Learn how to process your emotions by writing them down. Don't worry about grammar or bad penmanship; just get the words down on paper. Using the phrase "I feel... because...," write lots of pages about your feelings. Or take an emotional journey and keep a travelogue of your progress by recording "Today, I felt...." Journal writing has no rules. You can use a bound book with colored pages or simply scribble your feelings on pieces of paper. Don't get hung up on following a specific order or structure with your writing. Use whatever method feels right for you. Journal writing should be completely free-flowing, with no concerns about what someone would think about your words. You may want to store your journal in a private place or ask others to respect your privacy.

The torn-up letter. If you've used this method in the past, you know how effective it is. Record your thoughts and emotions as if you were writing a letter to someone. Then tear the letter up, burn it, or (if it's a short letter) even flush it down the toilet. You can also write your thoughts out in a temporary e-mail, then permanently delete your message.

Did It Work?

How do you know if expressing your emotions worked? You won't always know the answer right away. But don't let that stop you. What's important about expressing your feelings is that you *do* it.

Regardless of which methods you use, keep processing your feelings instead of bottling them up. Once you express what you feel, ask yourself, "Do I still want to *eat* that feeling?" If so, use a different method and try it again.

Continue to learn about emotions. Read books, talk to a counselor, or take classes to study issues like grief or anger. Keep practicing until expressing your emotions becomes second nature. Whenever you feel a strong or uncomfortable emotion, reach for a pen, seek a hug, or pull out your favorite CD instead of hunting for a bag of chocolate chip cookies.

CHAPTER SEVEN
What Do I Need?

HAVE YOU EVER HEARD AN OLD SONG on the radio and suddenly remembered a person or an event you hadn't thought about in years? Maybe it reminded you of your first love, a great concert, or a fun party. Just like that familiar old song, your favorite foods can also be connected to situations from your past.

Foods often become embedded in your memory, not just because of how they taste, but because of the feelings you originally had around them. Each time you associate a particular food with an event or an experience, you create a link that continues to exist, even years later.

Heather discovered an interesting connection between her childhood memories and her current struggles with craving popcorn.

I love popcorn. I don't just eat it for a snack, I practically binge on it. My parents were both alcoholics and when they'd been drinking, I would hide in my room because their yelling and fighting scared me. They pretty much got drunk every day, but for some reason they never drank on Sundays. I don't know if they wanted to start the week sober or what.

On Sunday evenings, I would sit on the couch between them and eat popcorn while we all watched TV. It was homemade popcorn, the old-fashioned kind with lots of salt and butter. Those evenings were one of the few times in my childhood I didn't feel afraid. Whenever I'm anxious or scared, I still reach for popcorn because it reminds me of feeling safe and secure.
—Heather

In today's world, emotional needs don't usually have easy solutions. We live miles away from our families, we worry about job stability, and we watch our friends move away to other states. It's easy to let food become a replacement for what we miss in our lives.

Food doesn't have to be the solution to your empty emotional places. You can learn how to take care of your needs in other ways. But before you can do this, you have to become clear on exactly what your needs are.

In this next step of conquering emotional eating, you'll learn how to identify and label the specific needs that make you want to eat. First, let's look again at how your needs and food became so connected.

The Food/Needs Connection

Sometimes you crave a specific food because it reminds you of getting your needs met in the past. Suppose you're at a baseball game and you get an overwhelming desire for a hot dog. Is it because you love the taste of hot dogs? Or is it because you love the *feelings* stirred by memories of fun times when you attended ball games as a child?

We tend to miss the happiness and comfort of good times in our past. But since we can't go back there, food becomes as close as we get. By eating a memory-associated food, we attempt to recapture those wonderful old feelings.

FOOD MEMORIES

Your memories related to specific foods often provide clues to how they meet your needs today. See if you can remember times in your childhood when you ate some of your favorite foods. Recall where you were and the people you were with at those times. The examples below might help you pull up your own food memories.

You can take this a step further by identifying how your emotional needs became linked to a specific food. By tracing back to your earliest recollections of eating a food, you can identify the needs that were met at that time. When you crave that food now, you might be experiencing the same needs as in your food memory.

Repeat this food tracing exercise for any other foods that contribute to your eating struggles. Any time you crave a specific food, see if you can match your current emotional needs to the ones in your food tracing. You might be amazed at how your favorite foods got hooked into meeting your needs.

Food	Emotional Need
Ice cream cones	Saturday night. We made a special trip into town and bought ice cream to celebrate the end of a week.
Red licorice	The local candy store. Mom let me go by myself and I got to choose what I wanted.
Pink cotton candy	Annual trip to the circus. It was one of the few times Dad and I went to an event by ourselves.
Three-layer chocolate cake	My birthday. I got to pick out the cake. A rare time when I felt noticed and valued.
Christmas pudding	Holiday gatherings, feeling cozy and happy.

Matching foods and needs. Food tracings help you recognize the connections between your unmet needs and the foods from your past. By correlating your food craving with a previous emotional response, you can instantly identify what you're missing or what you need at present.

What Is a Need?

In the context of emotional eating, the word "need" describes a want or a desire. Maybe you yearn for things that would make your life better—more time or money or even more people to do things with. Some of your needs might relate to wanting more attention, appreciation, or love.

Emotional needs come in all levels, from being bored or stressed to complex issues such as wanting to find a new relationship or

Food Tracing

Choose a favorite food (e.g., chocolate ice cream, coconut cake) that triggers you to overeat. Focusing on your childhood, think back to events or situations where you ate this food. You might remember family celebrations, certain friends, or perhaps lonely or difficult periods of life.

Try to recall one of your earliest memories associated with eating this food. Picture the scene in detail. Where are you? Who else is there? What emotions do you sense as you're eating? Are you feeling warm, comforted, safe, nurtured? Was this a time when your family was happy or peaceful? Maybe the food provided an escape from negative emotions like anger or fear. Notice whether your food memory is associated with grief or sadness.

Identify one or two of the strongest emotions that arise from your food memory and write down what you were feeling. Now think about your present struggle with this trigger food. When you crave it most, you may be longing for the emotions or people you've just identified in your food tracing.

Cookies = Feeling Safe

At my small country school in rural South Dakota, I struggled a lot with feeling awkward and not fitting in with the other kids. On cold, snowy days, I remember coming home to freshly baked cookies cooling on the kitchen table. My brother and I would drink glasses of milk and eat half a dozen cookies. Mom liked to bake, so she was usually very cheerful on those days. Sitting in that cozy kitchen made me feel warm, nurtured, and, most of all, very safe.

I've learned that when I start craving cookies, I'm usually feeling anxious or uneasy about something such as my work or other people's expectations. Eating cookies makes me feel confident, secure and emotionally safe. —Linda Spangle

make peace with a family member. Needs generally fall into one of three categories:

- **Simple needs:** Pleasure, fun, feeling better, stress relief
- **People needs:** Connecting, pleasing others, attention, appreciation
- **Emotional needs:** Love, nurturing, reward, safety, comfort, avoiding painful feelings

As you think about your own life, look for situations that you wish were different. Are you missing people? Do you need more money? Would you love to find new activities or events you could enjoy? Are there things in your life that you'd love to change or eliminate?

Emotional needs leave you with an emptiness and a longing to fill that need. When that doesn't happen, it's easy to let food do it for you. Lots of emotional eating struggles center around needing *something.* After you eat to fill the emotional holes, you feel better and you tend to forget about the needs. But when they pop back up, you have to look for food again. Instead of eating to fill those empty spots, it's time to discover other ways to meet your needs.

SIMPLE NEEDS

Simple needs are easy to spot and the solutions are fairly obvious. When you're bored, you look for activity; when you're tired, you take a nap. But simple needs can also make you grab food because it's a quick fix and doesn't require much effort. Here are some common simple needs that can prompt you to eat.

Pleasure, fun, and entertainment. Food gives us something to do! It entertains us with no strings attached, has no ulterior motives, and requires nothing in return. If you can't find anything you like on TV, you can always raid the refrigerator until the programs change.

With food, you don't have to wait for the fun to begin. You start getting enjoyment and satisfaction with the very first bite of a cookie or candy bar. On rainy afternoons or long weekends with no plans, food fills the empty hours. Putting food in your mouth makes the world more bearable. Later, when the painful realities of your life return, you simply eat again. For Jerry, food provided an escape from the drudgery of his life.

White Cake Frosting = Nurturing

My mother rarely praised me or approved anything I did. But my birthday was always a special occasion, and I got to skip my chores and pick what I wanted for dinner. For dessert, Mom would make a huge chocolate cake and frost it with thick, white icing. She made a big deal out of serving the cake and praising me for being the birthday girl. While I loved the birthday cake, I especially liked the smooth, creamy frosting. Because it was one of the few times I really felt noticed, I connected that frosting with nurturing and attention from my mother. I still get cravings for that type of homemade cake, although I often don't even eat the cake, just the frosting. Somehow the frosting still makes me feel nurtured and comforted. —Joyce

---

Macaroni and Cheese = Fun and Laughter

When I was eight years old, my younger brother died, and soon after that my mother started having severe migraine headaches. For years, we tiptoed around the house because she couldn't tolerate any type of noise. My father got depressed and usually spent evenings watching TV with a six-pack of beer. Once a week, our neighbor Margie invited me and my sister over for dinner, and she often served casseroles like macaroni and cheese. Margie's husband told funny stories and we could laugh as loud as we wanted without worrying about Mom's headaches. Now, when life gets too serious and hard, I start longing for macaroni and cheese because it helps me lighten up and feel like laughing again. —Roger

Lots of times, I eat just to put something in my face. It helps me stop thinking about how much I hate my life. I work in a dead-end job, my marriage is awful, and my kids are always in trouble. We constantly struggle with money, barely covering our bills each month. Most days, food is the only thing I have to look forward to. It's all I've got. —Jerry

Eating is quicker and easier than trying to invent new ways to entertain yourself or to cope with life. Jerry admits, "Without food, I'd have no fun at all!"

Security. When you feel anxious or afraid, eating gives you stamina and boosts your courage. If you feel nervous or uncomfortable at a party, you can just hide your feelings behind a plate of appetizers. When uneasiness creeps back in, you can simply eat more. Food becomes the security blanket that gets you through the evening.

When challenges affect your confidence, eating boosts your courage. Perhaps you eat a snack before presenting your big project at work. Or you grab a few cookies before calling your ex-husband about the child-support payments. As long as you have food, you feel strong enough to deal with your issues.

Transition. Have you noticed how food provides a convenient way to move from one event or time of day to another? Doughnuts start a meeting. Dessert ends a meal. Ice cream signifies bedtime. Even your late afternoon snack indicates you're home from work and ready to start your evening.

But what if your "food transition" is contributing to your weight gain? After a stressful work day, Kevin decided to stop at McDonald's on the way home. The next day, he did it again. Before he knew it, he'd slipped into the habit of going through the drive-up lane every day after work. After a year of "transition" snacks of french fries and milkshakes, Kevin had gained more than fifty pounds.

To break the pattern of using food for transition, you may need to shake up your routine. Drive home from work on a new street or turn into your driveway from the opposite direction. If you normally enter your house through the garage, switch to the front door, then immediately walk upstairs or into your den instead of toward the kitchen.

Invent new ways to mark transitions in your day. You can symbolize the end of your work day by drinking hot tea or a diet soda. Change your bedtime routine to include relaxing music or stretching exercises in place of a bowl of ice cream.

Procrastination. Food provides an excellent excuse for putting off the things you don't want to do. Suppose you need to mow the lawn or clean the house. It's easy to think, "I'll eat something first, then I'll get started." You might do the same thing with an important project at work or a school assignment. The larger or more difficult the job, the more times you'll eat to avoid it. Of course, after you finish your food, your distasteful task will still be waiting for you.

Sometimes eating helps avoid thinking. Food keeps you occupied and prevents you from focusing on the real issues in your life.

Christine's husband was a strong, domineering person who preferred to avoid discussions about serious issues. Christine knew for months that her marriage was in trouble, but she just couldn't face the discussion that would happen once she brought up the subject of getting a divorce. So whenever she contemplated talking to her husband, she would go to the refrigerator and get something to eat so she wouldn't have to think about it.

PEOPLE NEEDS

Food provides a universal string that connects us to others. Business deals, family reunions, even first-time dates typically include a meal. Having a plate of food in front of us puts us at ease in almost any situation. Whether we are with family, friends, or new coworkers, sharing a meal helps us relate to the people around us.

Connecting or belonging. Some days, sticking with your diet plan feels a lot harder than simply matching the way others eat. So at a restaurant, you join the group in ordering drinks and appetizers. And if the people you're with decide to eat dessert, you have one too. Eating the same as everyone else feels easier than standing out from the group.

Be careful about dropping your diet plan for the sake of connecting in a relationship. Every Saturday morning, Robin met a friend at a local coffee shop, where they'd catch up on the week's events. Often her friend would debate whether or not to order a doughnut. Because she wanted to feel close to her friend, Robin typically gave in and said, "If you want a doughnut, I'll have one with you."

Sometimes your efforts to connect don't work. After a disappointing date or a dull party, you may still yearn to feel close to people. Even chatting on the Internet can leave you feeling lonely and unsatisfied once you sign off. Heading to the refrigerator might seem like a good solution, but food can't make up for the absence of good companionship or meaningful conversations.

People-pleasing. Most of us don't like conflict, so when someone tells us to eat, we do. We get caught up in pleasing other people, even when that means eating a lot more than we want. Resisting could mean dealing with someone who feels insulted or hurt. Do any of these comments sound familiar?

"What's the matter, don't you like my food? I thought this was your favorite!"
"I made this cherry pie just for you. What do you mean you don't want any?"
"Come on, everyone else is eating. Besides, we have to celebrate!"

Families often have unspoken expectations regarding food. At family gatherings, people may expect you to stuff yourself with pasta or a huge grilled hamburger because "this is how we always eat." Once you give in, you may conclude it wasn't your fault. "What was I supposed to do? They begged me to join them and I didn't want to hurt their feelings."

When you eat because it's "expected," you give power to someone else instead of making your own decisions about your body. This ultimately damages your self-esteem as well as your weight.

For years, I endured the glares and snide comments from my husband's relatives whenever I tried to lose weight. Usually, I'd just give in and take second helpings and eat dessert along with everyone else. One day, it hit me that by eating to please my in-laws, I was giving them a lot of power. I got angry as I thought about all the years I'd sacrificed my weight-loss goals to keep peace in the family. So I made a decision that I would take care of myself and my needs instead of eating to please them. It took a while, but eventually they stopped pushing me to eat the way they did. —Barbara

Blaming others. Wouldn't it be nice if being overweight wasn't really your fault? You could simply explain that you have a weight problem because your mother (or boyfriend or boss) always insists that you eat. But it doesn't work that way. Any time you say, "I couldn't help it," what you really mean is "I didn't want to help it." And when you eat to avoid hurting people's feelings, you hurt yourself instead. While blaming someone else for your weight problem might sound legitimate, it simply allows you to avoid taking responsibility for your own actions.

Whenever I fell off my diet, I'd always blame other people—my friends, my family, my coworkers. I convinced myself "they" were the reason I failed. Finally I realized that no one was going to do this for me. I had to face my problems honestly and figure out how to make my plan work. —Pam

"It's not my fault." Sometimes we use food as a way to get a break from the demands of life. But rather than admit we simply want to eat, we create excuses to justify our behavior. Do any of these sound familiar?

- I was on vacation or out of town.
- I had people visiting me.
- It was my birthday.
- It was my husband's birthday.
- My mother is sick.

Who came up with the rule that you have to eat cake for everyone's birthday? If your mother is ill, does that mean you can't take care of yourself? These excuses make as much sense as trying to talk your way out of a speeding ticket by blaming the person who was tailgating you.

Birthdays and vacations. You don't have to compromise your eating goals just because someone becomes a year older. Instead of automatically joining birthday celebrations, become selective about which people you will eat cake for. You might decide to skip it for anyone who isn't a relative or for any children under the age of six. Or you can honor the birthday individual by eating a few bites of cake instead of a whole piece.

Here's a way to make a little game out this. At birthday celebrations, cut off a piece of cake about two inches square. Plan to take the final bite of your cake at the same time the last person in the group finishes eating. If you're at a gathering with small children, this can take a long time. You may have to be very patient as you wait for them to stop playing and finish their cake.

You might also consider taking a new approach to how you celebrate your own birthday. Sue decided to stop using her birthday as an excuse for having too much food and alcohol.

During the entire day of my birthday, I intentionally do things that will enhance my health and well-being, not shorten my life. I take time to exercise, I eat extra healthy and I don't eat cake or dessert. I may treat myself to a massage or a manicure. At the end of my self-care day, I usually feel great instead of depressed about being a year older. —Sue

You can do the same thing with a vacation. Instead of throwing away your rules about eating, define a vacation as a chance to take care of yourself.

When I go on vacation, I celebrate having time to exercise and actually pay attention to my eating. Rather than keeping my old habits of overindulging in food and alcohol, I relax by meditating and listening to music. By using a trip to renew myself, I don't end up needing another vacation to recover from the one I was on. —Nicki

EMOTIONAL NEEDS

Most people have a long list of emotional needs that aren't being met. We yearn for more love, attention, and affection. We crave nurturing, comfort, recognition, and reward. Many days, we struggle to cope with stress or depression or low self-esteem. As you explore your emotional needs, continue to look for ways to take care of yourself without using food to fill the holes in your life.

Eating as a reward. At the end of a hard day, you may feel you deserve a reward for your efforts. But in fact, no one even seems to notice your efforts. You simply want to be noticed and appreciated. When no one acknowledges your efforts, you feel empty and disappointed. So you reward yourself—by eating.

For many people, food as a reward started in childhood. Maybe you were told, "Be good and I'll give you a treat." Perhaps you've set up your own reward system. By promising yourself that you can eat afterwards, you motivate yourself to clean up the yard or study for an exam. You may even convince yourself you "deserve" food because of what you accomplished or the efforts you made.

But rewarding yourself with food is a hollow victory. In reality, you would much rather be noticed by the people you worked so hard to please. If only your boss would commend your work or your spouse would express appreciation, maybe you wouldn't feel so compelled to reach for a food reward.

Eating as an escape. As a hospital psychotherapist, Carla spent long days in intense counseling sessions with her clients. In addition to keeping up on paperwork and attending committee meetings, she supervised new therapists on staff. Much of the time, she raced from one office or appointment to another feeling she didn't have time to breathe between activities.

One afternoon, as she crammed down a candy bar, Carla noticed how calm she felt while she was eating. She said, "For a few seconds, my brain focused on my mouth instead of the other thoughts flying through my head. It was like getting a respite in the middle of my crazy day."

In our busy, chaotic lives, sometimes we want a break from all of our demands and responsibilities. When we eat, we tell our hectic thoughts, "Leave me alone for a little while! I'm eating!"

Eating to avoid feeling. When life is too painful, you can shove your struggles away by eating a whole pizza or another piece of chocolate cake. By literally swallowing your negative emotions, you can pretend you are over them or even deny they ever existed.

My friend Joyce was overwhelmed by grief and sadness when her fifteen-year marriage ended. She told me, "I can't bear what I'm going through. Isn't there some way to skip this part?"

Sorry, but you can't skip emotions. Unresolved grief or anger will eventually push to the surface, forcing you either to deal with the painful feelings or shove them back down with more food. For years, Monica tried to run from her grief, but it never quite worked.

After my twin brother died, I couldn't face the horrible pain I felt from losing him. So I decided to ignore my grief and simply not allow it in my life. But it was as though my emotions were stored in a huge box. Whenever I tried to lose weight, the box would peek open and the grief feelings would start to seep out. So I'd immediately eat until I shoved the lid back down. I finally realized that until I faced my grief and dealt with my emotional pain, I would never be successful with managing my weight. —Monica

Often, emotional needs are quite obvious and easy to identify. But sometimes you won't be able to figure out what you're missing or what you want. Is your need physical or emotional? Will a nap be enough or do you need a vacation? Perhaps you want time alone but you also need to find new friends. Some days lots of emotional needs will be circling at the same time. Your job is to learn how to identify these needs so you can take the next step of doing something about them without reaching for food.

Gathering Your Needs

A number of years ago, a local weight-loss counselor promoted his business using refrigerator magnets that read, "It's not in here!" It's true that whatever you need, it's NOT in the refrigerator. But before you can resolve your needs in ways that don't involve food, you need to become skilled at knowing exactly what you're trying to fix.

Gary works full-time as a clinical director at a major psychiatric hospital. Most evenings, he also sees patients in his private counseling practice. Between the two, he fights traffic, grabs a quick meal, and tries to figure out how to spend a few minutes with his wife and his five children. Weeks go by without Gary having an hour to himself. His life is filled meeting work demands and taking care of other people.

Gary says, "I don't know how my life got so out of hand. My days fly by, but I never get caught up with all my tasks. I feel like I'm missing a lot of things and I suspect I'm using food to replace them." When Gary made a list of his needs, here is what he came up with.

- Time: I wish I wasn't always behind and trying to get caught up.
- Closeness: More intimacy with my wife, feeling closer to my kids.
- Connection: Time with people who are authentic, encouraging, and not so demanding.
- Meaning: I'd like to watch TV programs that show something other than violence or shallow relationships.
- Fun: More enjoyment out of life, not so burdened by all my required activities.
- Hope: See the potential for life to get better instead of being so pessimistic about it.

• Feel settled: Instead of feeling restless and constantly searching for meaning and peace.

As he reviewed his list, Gary began to understand what food was doing for him. It was taking the place of everything he yearned for but didn't have.

YOUR NEEDS LIST

As you think about your own needs, you may find some of them don't fit neatly into any categories. What's important is that you take time to look for them and learn how to address them creatively. Here's an exercise to help you identify what you need.

Find a quiet place where you can be alone and focus on your thoughts without being interrupted. If you wish, you can also tape record your needs, then write them down later or ask another person to write your list as you do this exercise.

At the top of a blank piece of paper write the question "What do I need?" Focusing on the present moment as well as life in general, think about where you are lacking or missing something. Take a few deep breaths to relax, then ask yourself, "What do I need?"

Using one or two words or short phrases, make a list of all the needs you can think of. Consider needs related to your weight, self-esteem, stress, job, or relationship issues as well as personal concerns. Include simple needs like money or rest and complex ones like a new job or a different life partner. Don't worry about providing explanations or long descriptions right now, just make a simple list of what you need. If you get stuck, keep asking yourself, "What *else* do I need?"

When you can't think of any more needs, picture a brick wall in front of you. Notice a long crack running all the way from the top of the wall to the bottom. In your mind, step forward and push on the crack until the wall opens enough for you to walk through. Take a minute to picture the scene in front of you. Than ask the question again, "What do I need?"

Allow whatever thoughts come to you, then write down those additional words. When you feel completely finished and nothing more comes to mind, mentally step back through the wall. Picture the sections closing together and the crack disappearing, leaving a solid brick wall. Relax a few minutes to help you feel calm and centered.

When you finish, read through the needs you identified. Most likely, your initial list will include needs like nurturing, less stress, more money, etc. But you may find that once you mentally pushed through the brick wall, your list of needs began to shift. Here you may find words like safety, affirmation, intimacy, or perhaps escape.

At some point, find a place where you can read your list out loud. Notice how it feels to hear yourself speaking about what you need in your life. Don't be surprised if this exercise brings tears to your eyes. You may have gone a long time without acknowledging what you truly need and want in your life. Or you may have buried your needs for the sake of taking care of others. If you don't believe you can get your needs met, you may even have avoided thinking about them.

If you have trouble identifying what you need, use the list on page 134 to prompt some ideas. Don't get hung up saying "I can't do anything about that!" Right now, your task is to identify exactly what is contributing to your emotional eating. You won't be able to fix all of these needs right away, but knowing what they are will help you recognize where to start making changes.

Reviewing your needs. You can do the exercise "What do I need?" anytime and anywhere. Although it might be helpful, you don't always have to write your needs down. You could men-

Common Needs

Simple

Adventure
Cleaner house
Fun
Go dancing
Input, education
Less boredom
Listen to music
Love
Money

More exercise
New hobby
New house
New or different job
Project to work on
Read
Rest
Time
Vacation

People

Closeness to family
Belong to group
Meet new people
Community involvement
Get along better with others
Kindness from others
More close friends
People to have fun with

Someone to share hobbies with
Stimulating discussions
Learning relationships
More intimacy
Different partner, lover, spouse
Patience with others
Stop pleasing others
Break from being with people

Emotional

Affection
Appreciation
Approval
Attention
Calm
Comfort
Feel better about myself
Feel less burdened
Feel safe

Fewer demands
Hope
Less stress
Love
Meaning in life
Nurturing
Peace
Validation

tally list your needs while driving to work or waiting for an appointment.

Repeat this exercise at intervals. While some of your general needs will stay the same, other ones change from day to day. Identifying what you need won't always stop you from emotional eating, but it will help you see the connection between having a need and using food to fulfill it for you. When Kaye listed her needs, she was able to understand why she struggled so much with emotional eating.

I miss a lot of things I used to have in my life. I wish I had time to sit outside under a tree and read a good book. I miss being held, making those special dinners, being appreciated, having a slow day.

But since I can't seem to get those things, I reach for food instead. A bag of chips or cookies replaces the bubbly home I wish I had. Snacks in my work drawer fill in for the compliments I'm not getting. The bowl of ice cream late at night takes the place of arms around me. —Kaye

Getting What You Need

How do you change your eating patterns when your needs are so great and food is so easy? When you can't find a minute to yourself during the day, where do you start? As hard as it is, you have to be willing to take charge of your own life, including taking time for yourself. This may require moving yourself up on your priority list, ahead of your aging mother or your demanding boss.

Getting your needs met doesn't require changing your entire life at once. Many of your needs can be handled by doing a simple action or even changing your thinking. Try the following exercise to get you started.

Take out the list of needs you wrote earlier. Feel free to add to it, focusing on what you want in life right now, today, or even this very moment. You can also write a new list that's specific to a situation, like managing your job, dealing with a current relationship, or coping with a visit with your parents.

Be sure you've written "What do I need?" above your list. Now add a column to the other side of your paper and at the top, write "How could I get it?"

For each item on your list, identify what it would take to get that specific need met, even partially, and record your answers. Consider every possible solution that would help appease your emotional needs, at least long enough to keep you out of the refrigerator.

Remember Gary's list? Many of his needs related to his current job and the pressures of his finances and his family life. He knew that, eventually, he wanted to find a lower-stress job closer to his home. But in the meantime, he had to make some changes that would meet his needs right now. Gary's list is shown below.

What do I need?	How could I get it?
Time	Limit my private practice to two nights a week, no exceptions
Closeness	Set up a date night with my wife, develop bedtime rituals with the kids
Connection	Plan lunch with my favorite professor from graduate school
Meaning	Skip TV; play games with kids or read instead
Fun	Listen to my opera CDs during my commute
Hope	Talk with my wife about our long-term plans
Feel settled	Slow down, live more in the present moment

Within a week, Gary felt more in charge of his life again and began to investigate how he could make other changes as well. "Doing those simple things took away a lot of the food cravings I'd been fighting for so long. Instead of eating to make my life go away, I discovered I had the power to heal my own pain."

Make It Happen

When you create solutions that will meet your needs, make them happen. Take a walk, close your office door, hug your child. Often one simple action will redirect how you manage your entire day. What seemed so overwhelming that you had push it away with food suddenly becomes more bearable.

You can use exercises in this chapter in many ways, from thinking about life in general to focusing on a very specific problem or event. When you wake up in the morning, ask yourself, "What do I need today?" If you're going to a party or visiting your mother, consider the question, "What do I need during this specific time?"

Jack Canfield, coauthor of the *Chicken Soup for the Soul* series, suggests adding the question, "What is the experience or emotion I'm looking for?" As you seek ways to meet your needs, this question prompts you to look even further. For example, when you want attention or affirmation, asking your partner for feedback may help meet that need. But at the same time, you might also be looking for intimacy and physical closeness.

It's Up to You

As much as you wish someone else would fix your life, ultimately you have to fix it yourself. Even if you believe your family or boss or lover "should" do more for you, others can never fill all the gaps in your life. It's up to you to figure out how to get your needs met.

You may find this difficult to accept. Perhaps you feel angry or resentful that people around you aren't doing their part to meet your needs. But you can waste a lot of energy and time being angry that the world isn't taking care of you. Instead of wishing other people would do more for you, look for creative ways to manage your needs by yourself.

CHANGE WHAT YOU CAN

When you feel overwhelmed by your needs, take a careful look at the demands and responsibilities in your life. If you keep piling on more obligations, eventually something will be shortchanged. Unfortunately, you may forgo basic needs such as rest, healthy eating, and stress relief and soon your self-care quietly slips away. Food takes a lot less time and effort than going to the gym or calling a friend.

Whenever you add something to your life, ask yourself, "What am I willing to take away?" Then decide if you can live with the answer. It may not be easy to eliminate things you enjoy or consider important. But if you don't make any changes, something will fall off the edge on its own. Usually it's your own needs that are sacrificed.

Take charge of your life. Any time you start searching for food when you know you aren't hungry, stop and ask yourself what you need. By taking a few minutes to identify what's behind your desire to eat, you postpone grabbing food and instead take care of what you really wanted in the first place.

CHAPTER EIGHT

Nurturing without Food

DO YOU EVER HAVE DAYS WHEN you feel emotionally exhausted, discouraged, or worn out? Nothing's really "wrong," but you feel so alone in your struggles. You wish you knew how to fix the empty spots in your life. If only you could be held, soothed, and appreciated. What you want more than anything is to be *nurtured*.

In our no-touch, hard-work society, nurturing has become almost nonexistent. In fact, most things in life are *not* nurturing. Budget meetings, traffic jams, crying kids, and preoccupied spouses can all leave you feeling raw and more alone than ever.

When you look for a way to ease your emotional burdens, food is often the first thing that comes to mind. Eating fills the gaps in your life. It renews your "empty places" and helps you forget the things or the people you are missing.

Food probably wouldn't be so attractive if you could find nurturing more easily. You keep hoping someone will care about how you're doing. "Maybe *this time,* someone will pay attention, call me, or hold me." But the phone doesn't ring, no one comes to the door, and everyone goes home to families—except *you.*

No wonder you go to the refrigerator! It holds such potential—the cool, soothing texture of ice cream, with just enough chocolate and nuts to make it entertaining. Maybe you find a creamy slice of cheesecake, a bit of leftover casserole, or some frozen cookie dough. You probably have your own list of foods that always seem to make you feel better.

But of course, food isn't the only option. Now that you know how to identify your needs, you are ready to build the skills for fulfilling those needs. In this chapter, you'll focus on meeting your needs for nurturing without using food. You'll also learn how to fill the emotional emptiness that results from boredom, restlessness, loneliness, and depression.

True nurturing heals your soul. When you've been nurtured well, you feel uplifted, comforted, and eased. Like being wrapped in a blanket and held tightly, nurturing makes you feel *safe*. When you know how to nurture yourself, you can create ways to feel comforted and secure, even in the midst of your hectic day.

Emotional Safety

If you're like most people, you carefully protect your physical safety. You buckle up in the car, lock your door at night, and stay out of the scary parts of town. But how do you protect your "emotional safety"? What do you do when life makes you unsettled, anxious, and insecure?

Self-care activities such as taking a warm bath or getting a massage can certainly help. But a sense of emotional safety forms the base for your nurturing efforts, making them more effective and satisfying. Being emotionally safe helps you feel grounded and confident that you can handle life's challenges. Like an invisible shield, emotional safety makes you feel protected, strong, and secure.

When you're in a good mood, life is going well, and you have no particular worries, emotional safety is probably not an issue. But when life wears you down and makes you uneasy or anxious, you may need to take steps to rebuild your feelings of safety. Here are some ways to help the process.

SLOW DOWN!

Emotional safety doesn't happen fast. Racing from one thing to the next, barely leaving yourself time to take a breath does *not* make you feel settled or strong. So learn to slow down and pay attention to things around you. Focus on small, unexpected joys that life brings you—a fragrant flower, a cool evening breeze, a hot cup of tea.

Once in a while, take a break from your demands and center yourself by "holding still" inside your mind. Take a few deep breaths, then gaze quietly at the sky or some other aspect of nature. Focus on the vibrant colors of trees or flowers. Notice the cloud formations or the rocks and dirt that form a walking path. Instead of reaching for something to eat, use this mental release to bring you back to emotional safety.

Noise is not nurturing. Listening to loud music or talking with lots of people can be fun, but these things aren't necessarily going to make you feel nurtured. When you want to feel emotionally safe, seek out and appreciate quiet. If you usually go to bustling, noisy restaurants, look for a few that have a soothing, calm atmosphere. At home, take time to close your eyes, play soft music, and allow your spirit to feel renewed.

CREATE SAFE PLACES

When you outgrew your pacifier as a child, you probably looked for something else to make you feel safe and content. Maybe you slept with a ragged blanket or a beat-up stuffed animal in your bed.

But where are the "teddy bears" in your life today? While you may have outgrown your toys, sometimes you still need an emotional "security blanket."

In your home or your work setting, find a room or a corner that you can turn into a safe place. In this special area, surround yourself with favorite objects that make you feel secure and comfortable. Personalize the room, if you want, by adding more posters, candles, or stuffed animals.

Brighten your mood with a few plants, either live ones or authentic-looking silk arrangements. Keep a variety of CDs in your car for easing your tension at the end of the day. If you go to a lot of meetings, carry a favorite coffee cup with you. It will give you something familiar to hold on to, especially during tense discussions.

Whenever I relocated my office through the years, right away I started to make the new place emotionally safe. I moved my desk and chairs around until the space "felt right." I placed stuffed animals on the bookcases, picked the best walls for my favorite pictures, and arranged my plants in the corners next to the windows.

I usually knew when I had it right. The room felt warm, cozy, and very safe. Although I still had to learn which streets to avoid during rush hour, once I got inside my office, I felt confident that I could handle my work.

Like the soldiers who decorate a twig with tiny lights and call it a Christmas tree, you can create emotional safety anywhere. If you start a new job or move to a different home, don't wait for months to "fix things up." Take steps immediately to make yourself feel comfortable and at ease, even in a brand-new setting.

Search out areas you can use as an oasis or a safe retreat, even in the midst of chaos. The bathtub, a nearby park, your car, even a neighborhood coffee shop can all become safe places to hide and regroup when you need it.

Develop Rituals and Routines

You can also build emotional safety by creating rituals that help you feel more settled or organized. Think for a minute about your daily routines. How do you organize yourself for the day? Do you always start by getting a cup of coffee or making the rounds and greeting your friends? When you get home, do you typically sit down and read the mail for a few minutes?

Rituals make you feel safe because you do the same things each time rather than constantly having to face or think up something new. Look at the patterns you already have in place. If your daily rituals always include food, you may have to create some new routines to conquer your emotional eating.

As a newspaper journalist, Jamie was under constant pressure to research and complete her news stories before press deadlines. To wind down after a hectic day, she usually snacked on chips and candy bars on the way home from work. When she joined a new weight-loss program, Jamie decided to change her afternoon rituals.

Now I stop at the park every day to appreciate the trees, talk to the squirrels, and mentally relax from my work. I sit on a bench and write in my journal, then lay out my plans for the evening. By slowing down and soothing my emotional soul, I'm able to handle the demands of my family without feeling like I have to eat something before I can face them.—Jamie

If you tend to use food to nurture yourself, start creating new rituals you can follow instead of eating. You might want to develop ones for different times of day or aspects of your life. For example, plan one routine for after work and another for times when you spend an evening by yourself. Here are a few ideas.

• Listen to a particular song or type of music such as a favorite classical piece.

- Light candles and sit quietly or meditate for a while before starting dinner.
- Read a few pages from a book of poetry, a novel, or the Bible.
- Put your feet up and spend a few minutes reading the mail or the newspaper.
- Have a cup of tea or coffee along with a planned, healthy snack.
- Listen to quiet, instrumental music each night before you drift off to sleep.

When you travel, decide how to make yourself feel "at home" in a hotel room or someone else's house. Tuck your favorite slippers into your suitcase or bring photos of your loved ones to place on a bedside stand. Rather than be disappointed because a restaurant doesn't carry your favorite tea, keep a few packets of your favorite ones in your purse.

How to Nurture Yourself

Do you ever look forward to going home for a holiday or weekend because you're hoping someone will take care of you? After all, your home should be the one place you can count on for nurturing. But lots of times that doesn't happen, and you leave feeling angry, disappointed, and let down.

Of course, nothing replaces getting a warm hug or a few encouraging words from those you love. It would be so nice if other people would always provide the support and comfort you need. But in reality, you're on your own. Instead of waiting for someone else to be there for you, turn the tables and learn to be there for *yourself*.

Doing all of your own nurturing isn't always easy or enjoyable, but it beats not getting your needs met. It also helps you accept people for who *they* are, and understand why they may not be able to nurture you right when you need it, instead of constantly wishing they were different.

Melanie couldn't figure out what was wrong. The last few times she'd gone home for a weekend, she ate almost the entire time she was visiting. As she sat at the table trying to converse with her mother, she kept reaching for a few more homemade cookies or another piece of cake.

Ever since her father became ill, Melanie's mom had become distant and preoccupied. Whenever the discussion centered on someone else's problems, she couldn't seem to stay focused and would soon change the subject. Melanie resented the fact that she couldn't get any nurturing or attention from her mother or the rest of her family.

I think I came home holding an "electrical cord" that needed an energy charge to help me cope with my problems. In the past, when I plugged into my home, everything worked fine. But this time, nothing happened. Finally, I realized the power source was gone. The outlet looked fine on the outside, but behind the wall, the wires were so thin that hardly any power could get through.

Once I understood that my family couldn't meet my needs any more, I decided to look elsewhere for my energy boost. So I started doing more things to take care of myself. I also changed my expectations about my trips home. Instead of waiting for my parents to nurture me, I tried to listen to them more and stopped judging them so harshly. I also looked for ways to let them plug into me and draw off of my energy. My efforts didn't change the situation but they changed my attitude, and my visits home became a lot more enjoyable.—Melanie

Over time, Melanie developed ways to feel nurtured without depending on her family. Instead of sitting in the kitchen eating cookies, she took lots of walks and spent more time outdoors. At night she drove into the country to look at the stars away from the city lights. She wrote in her journal, hugged her mother a lot, meditated, and drank herb teas that she brought from home. By taking charge of her own nurturing, Melanie was also able to stop all of her extra eating.

Self-nurturing doesn't have to be complicated or time consuming. It only takes a few minutes to do something that makes you feel better. As you work on self-nurturing, decide what helps you most when you need to feel comforted or relaxed. Build a mental toolbox of things that work, perhaps even matching specific ones to different settings or times of day.

Ideally, most of your nurturing actions should not be food related. However, if chatting with your best friend over lunch makes you feel nurtured and cared for, keep that activity on your list. You don't have to completely avoid food as a source of nurturing; just make sure eating is only a minor part of your efforts. When you depend on food itself to make you feel better, you've slid back into emotional eating.

Draw on What You Love

Use this next exercise ("What I Love") to help you plan your nurturing activities. Before you begin, take a few minutes to think about what you love. In addition to your favorite methods of relaxation or stress relief, consider everything that *energizes you, gives you joy, or fills you with delight.*

Post the list where you can see it easily. Each day, select at least one item and use it to nurture yourself. Sometimes you can feel nurtured by simply doing one tiny thing that takes you out of your ordinary daily routine and gives you a sense of fun or satisfaction. Think of these things as gifts to yourself, a celebration of being "you."

What I Love

Take out a piece of paper and write the words "What I Love" at the top of the page. Then start writing. List everything you can think of that matches that description. Include people, activities, pets, and meaningful things such as sunsets or green grass. Don't spend a long time thinking about this—simply write down everything you consider nurturing, even if some of the items aren't always available or accessible.

Here are a few categories to get you started. Feel free to add others that fit for you.

- People, including friends, family, work colleagues
- Household pets as well as other animals such as horses
- Activities like sports, games, crafts, reading
- Events like concerts or plays, conferences, vacations
- Nature-related items like flowers, trees, gardens
- Familiar objects such as stuffed animals, pottery, photos
- Meaningful scenery like sunsets or starry nights
- Soothing, relaxing things such as a hot bath, massage, yoga

When you've completed your list, do a "six-month check" of everything on it. Put a check mark next to anything you haven't done, seen, or appreciated in the past six months. Use these marks to identify all the nurturing activities you've lost touch with or forgotten about. If your list includes seasonal things like skiing or gardening, simply keep them in mind for future planning.

Set a goal of going through everything on your list at least once, then starting again from the beginning. Don't worry about having your nurturing list in any particular order. If you want, you can separate it into categories later. But when you start doing things on your list, you might actually enjoy following the random order of how your ideas showed up.

Here are some examples from my own list of things I love: singing, my dogs, my family, sewing, gardening, riding my bike, good conversations, going to movies, reading, and dancing.

TAKE A RENEWAL WALK

When you feel worn out and disconnected from the world, you need to revive your spirit as well as your energy. Here's an instant renewal exercise that you can do in any setting.

Take a walk that is *not* designated as exercise. If you can't get outside, do your walk at a mall or even inside your office. For five to ten minutes, walk slowly and purposefully, with an openness to the world around you. Relax into your surroundings and mentally leave your problems and issues behind.

As you walk, focus on appreciating your five senses—sight, hearing, smell, taste, and touch. With each one, notice and experience things you might normally miss. Focus your eyes on something new; listen for sounds you hadn't realized were there. Smell and taste something different and notice the sensations. Touch a specific object and observe its texture and character.

Notice how you feel when you're finished. Did you get a sense of being relaxed and renewed? When you narrow your focus to include only your five senses, you shut out the rest of the world and give yourself a mini-nurturing break. With the simple act of connecting to your inner self, you can boost your energy and your confidence without needing to reach for food.

Nurturing Challenges

Many of your nurturing needs can be fixed with simple activities. But some issues are more subtle or not quite what they seem. Here are a few needs that, at first glance, might not appear to be related to nurturing.

BOREDOM

Saying "I'm bored" sounds so legitimate. When there's nothing on TV and no one to talk to, you pace the house, thinking you're bored. Soon you head to the refrigerator in search of entertainment. You defend yourself by saying "I didn't have anything to do, so I got something to eat."

But were you really dealing with boredom or did you need something else? Maybe you would have loved some companionship or a challenging activity. Instead of assuming you're bored, see if you can identify what might be missing in your life. You can separate boredom into different levels, then create slightly different solutions for each one.

Wanting something to do. This level is probably the closest to true boredom. When there's a gap in your life, you look for activity, diversion, entertainment—anything that would provide some fun or distraction. With this kind of boredom you don't have a big emotional need, you're just looking for the next item in life. When you can't come up with anything to do, it's easy to start looking for food.

If you watch a lot of TV, you may actually be adding to your boredom. Television is a passive form of entertainment and it rarely engages or challenges you mentally. It's easy to lie on the couch, surf the channels, and stare blindly at nonsense programming for hours on end. Using TV for nurturing is a setup for emotional eating.

To manage this level of boredom, create new diversion activities. Rent an unusual movie or pick up a new book. Get in touch with friends you haven't seen for a while or search the Internet for new subjects that would be fun to study.

Feeling bored when you don't have any planned activities can happen to anyone. We all occasionally have an evening or a weekend when there's not much going on. But if you tend to feel bored every night, you probably need to make some changes in your life instead of just looking for more entertainment.

Seeking experiences or meaning. Do you have a hard time getting your friends to make plans? Maybe you miss having a partner or family members around to do things with. Perhaps you wish you could feel more connected with people or find activities with meaning attached to them. Maybe you'd like to see a movie with an interesting friend, then discuss the plot over cappuccinos. Or you'd love to hear a classical music interpretation that would move you to tears.

With this level of boredom, you want more than just something to do. What you're actually searching for are "memory makers"—experiences that will provide lasting value. You want to remember the event and mentally re-live it the next day, thinking, "That was such a great time!"

When you feel this type of boredom, try reviving interests from your past or picking up some new skills. Maybe it's time to go back to sewing, crafts, astronomy, or chess. Perhaps you could start gardening or woodworking. You might be surprised at how much you enjoy crossword or jigsaw puzzles. Try your hand at creative writing projects such as poetry or short stories. Even writing your thoughts in a journal can relieve your boredom by helping you sort through your feelings and ideas.

Wanting a challenge. Does your life ever seem dull? Are the same old things going on every day? Maybe you'd give anything to rise above your daily routine and experience a higher level of excitement, newness, or personal growth. Even when you have lots of people to relate to, you may still feel empty and unfulfilled. You really want something to challenge or intrigue you, to make you feel excited about life again.

To resolve this level of boredom, explore things that are entirely new or different from your usual routine. Consider taking (or teaching) a class in a subject that interests you. Maybe you could study astronomy or participate in an archeological dig. Explore your hidden artistic skills by taking up oil painting or sculpture.

Challenge yourself to do small deeds of kindness that will make a difference in someone's life. Volunteer at a nursing home or tutor someone in reading or math. If you're physically capable of it, consider training for an athletic event, like an organized walk or a bike race. Find a personal trainer or rent videos and learn strength-training exercises.

Don't let boredom become an easy excuse for eating. Whenever you feel "bored," take a few minutes to determine exactly which type of boredom you are experiencing. If you feel trapped in your life situation, you're probably facing more than just boredom. Instead of using food as an easy way out, get out of the trap and make changes that address the bigger issue.

AFTER THE PARTY'S OVER

Have you ever followed your diet perfectly in a social setting, then overeaten later? This "after the party's over" eating can happen any time, but you may notice it most after you've attended a social event or a holiday celebration.

I've seen this pattern many times after big holidays like Thanksgiving or Passover. My clients carefully planned out the day, including eating a healthy breakfast and getting some exercise. Then they set up a detailed strategy for managing the holiday dinner itself.

Most of the time this worked fine and they got through the day without overeating. But on the day after the gathering, they started nibbling leftovers in the morning, then continued eating all day, sometimes even through the next week.

After you've managed an eating event exceptionally well, you may notice you get an "after the party's over" letdown. While you were resisting sampling all the desserts, you may have secretly resented that you couldn't eat like everyone else. If you don't work past these feelings, you tend to make up for them by overeating once you're alone.

When you attend a holiday dinner or a party, anticipate the let-down that can follow your heroic attempts to stay on your diet. Make plans for what you'll do in the hours *after* the event or the day *after* the holiday. Take an extra walk, call a friend for support, or plan self-nurturing activities that protect you from giving in to the "after the party's over" temptations.

When There Isn't Enough

Many years ago, I visited the home of my niece, Leah, who was six years old at the time. As I finished reading her bedtime story on the last night of my visit, Leah pleaded with me to stay longer. "Do you have to go home tomorrow? Can't you please stay here a few more days? Could you sleep in my room tonight?" I told her I'd love to stay but I had to return home the next day to go back to work. She started to cry and then begged, "Are you sure you can't stay a few more days or maybe for another week?"

Since this was unusual behavior for Leah, I wasn't sure how to respond. Leah's father had recently started a job in another city and was coming home only once a month. The rest of the family planned to move after school finished and their house sold. As I looked at Leah's sad little face, I said, "You miss your daddy, don't you?"

"Oh yes," she responded. "I miss him a lot. I wish he was here tonight." Then I asked her, "Leah, if I stayed sitting on your bed all night, would that be long enough? Or if I stayed at your house for another week, would that be enough? Because I think you're miss-ing your daddy a lot, and no matter how long I stay, you'll still wish he was here with you."

Leah nodded and tearfully admitted, "You're right. Even if you stayed here, my daddy would still be away. So I guess no matter how long you stay at our house, it won't be enough."

Many times we feel like we can't get *enough*. Even lots of hugs or compliments or salary raises don't seem to fill what we really need in our lives. Unfortunately, food works the same way. Some days, all of the food in the world won't be enough to solve your problems.

Whenever she had a hard time at work, Beth would eat until she got over the tension of her day. Finally, she recognized that food wasn't taking care of what she *really* needed.

Yesterday was a terrible day. My boss yelled at me, my computer crashed, and the phones never stopped ringing. On the way home, I stopped at the grocery store and bought a large bag of malted milk balls. I ate two of them before I left the store and about a dozen more once I got in the car. As I reached into the bag every few minutes while I was driving, I realized how silly this was. I asked myself, "How many malted milk balls will it take to make me feel better? Two? A dozen? A ton?" And I knew the answer. No matter how many I ate, there wouldn't be enough. So I stopped and threw the rest of the bag into the trash, then I went home to take care of myself.
—Beth

When you eat to fix emotional needs, it's like pouring water into a bucket with a hole in the bottom. No matter how much you put into it, the bucket will never get filled. A common saying in addiction treatment is "You can't get enough of what you don't really want." In the same way, eating more food when you actually need nurturing is not going to fill the emptiness you feel.

The "Emotional Cold"

Sometimes after weeks or even months of successfully managing your emotional eating, you'll hit a period where you let everything go. Perhaps you start feeling a little moody or discouraged or depressed. You just want to eat! A six-pack of beer and a large pizza magically appear in your living room. Or you start nibbling on the coffee cake and you keep going back to it until the pan is empty.

When this happens, don't give up or assume you've lost your skills. You may simply be suffering from an "emotional cold." For a brief period, this condition can decrease your ability to cope with life, prompting you to use food as a way to feel better. When you get an emotional cold, you can't usually talk yourself out of it, ignore it, or shake it off. You just have to wait until it gets better.

This "emotional cold" can be brought on by any number of stressful things—a struggling relationship, a job layoff, or just being sick of life at the moment. Maybe an unusual work challenge or an ill parent wore you out. Don't blame yourself or conclude that you're weak or a "failure." Instead, give yourself an emotional break and wait it out. Do lots of extra self-care and acknowledge yourself for your efforts to get better.

Take some time to heal from your "cold," then watch for signs that you're recovering. By viewing this period as just temporary "downtime," you aren't as likely to give up and slip back into your old emotional eating habits.

Once you've recovered, rebuild a sense of emotional safety, and return to your list of non-food ways to nurture yourself. As the years go by, you'll get better at protecting yourself from these emotional downtimes. But for now, simply focus on ways to "minimize the damage" and recover quickly.

As you practice the art of nurturing yourself, you will be amazed at how easy it is to take care of your own needs. You'll also discover that your favorite methods come to mind sooner, eventually replacing your thoughts of immediately reaching for food whenever you need to be nurtured.

CHAPTER NINE

What's in My Way?

"I KNOW WHAT TO DO, I just don't do it!"

How often have you said these words? If you're like most over-weight people, you can't blame your weight-loss failures on lack of knowledge. Despite all your good intentions, you just don't follow through on your promises to change your behavior.

For the past year, Shirley had been attending a weight-loss support group, but she'd made little progress in losing weight.

I constantly tell myself that I want to change, but nothing happens. I weigh exactly the same amount I did last year at this time. I still can't get myself into a consistent exercise program. And whether I want to admit it or not, food is still my very good friend. —Shirley

Thousands of dieters have a similar story. Your own bookshelf is probably filled with dieting guides and low-fat cookbooks, yet most days you never turn on your stove. You tell yourself that "one of these days" you'll start losing weight or working on your emotional eating problems. But you never quite get started.

So what's in your way? What keeps you from doing better self-care or expressing your feelings instead of eating to escape them?

More importantly, how can you quit stalling and start changing your life?

In this chapter, you'll face hard questions about what prevents you from dealing with your emotional issues. As you explore what's in your way, you'll find that many of these barriers affect other areas of your life as well. The same obstacles that keep you from nurturing yourself will also affect your exercise program and your ability to stay on your diet plan.

You don't have to let barriers stop you. If you're determined to change, start finding ways to get around the roadblocks that keep you stuck. Look at your excuses (because that's all they are) and start doing something about them instead of letting them get in the way of your progress.

Simple Barriers

Whenever you slip back into emotional eating, your first inclination is to explain why it wasn't your fault—you were way too busy, your sister is getting a divorce, or you had to work overtime. These sound like legitimate excuses. But did they really keep you from eating right or exercising?

These simple barriers don't involve a lot of psychological issues. But sometimes they're just enough to throw you off target and make you reach for food. When you hit simple barriers like being tired or getting a bad attitude, take a few quick actions to sidestep what's in your way instead of letting it get you into eating trouble.

"I'M TIRED! I'M BUSY! I'M STRESSED OUT!"

It's hard to work on your emotions when you're exhausted. So when you're too tired to focus on your self-care, get some sleep, then start again. When you wake up in the morning, lay out a new plan by creating a "What do I need?" list for the day.

Include words such as "rest" and "relaxing," then really think about how you can get those needs met. Could you set aside time to read a few pages of your novel or to catch a short nap? Do you need to eliminate a few demands so you can get some extra sleep?

When fatigue or stress start getting you down, grab a "slice of life" and tuck a self-care activity into a tiny segment of your day. Here are a few ideas that take only minutes to accomplish.

- Listen to a favorite song.
- Make a cup of herbal tea.
- Spend a few minutes with your pet.
- Light a candle and take ten deep breaths.
- Read a few low-fat recipes to get some ideas for planning healthy meals.

If you postpone taking care of yourself until you have enough time or energy, you'll probably never do it. So instead of waiting for a perfect time, learn how to slip a few miniature self-care activities into your daily life.

"I Don't 'Feel' Like It!"

Sometimes we just don't feel like doing things that take effort. We want what's easy, and eating is definitely easy. But to stop the pattern of reaching for an easy fix, you have to take care of yourself even when you *don't* feel like it.

Paul needed to lose over one hundred pounds. So he started a new diet plan, determined to stick with it until he reached his goal. Most days he felt strong with his program, but he admitted that once in a while he got discouraged and stopped caring.

Some days, I use the tools such as figuring out what I need and express-
ing what I feel, but it's not enough. My motivation slips and I don't care if
I eat right or not. Today, I sneaked over to the bakery and came back to my
office with a big piece of carrot cake. And was it ever good! But now, I wish
I had cared a little more before I gave in and ate it. —Paul

Even on a really bad day, don't stop caring. Tell yourself you are
worth it and you deserve to improve your life. After his carrot cake
episode, Paul vowed he would not stop caring, no matter what. So
he put a note on his computer where he would see it first thing
when he got to work. Every morning, he started his day by reading "I do care! I will always care! And I will make it!"

When you don't "feel" like facing your emotional needs, it's a
sign that something requires your attention. Dig beneath your
excuses and see what might be getting to you. Are you feeling
overwhelmed by resentment or anger? Has life been unfair lately?
Maybe you've been worn down by a string of difficult people or
stressful events. Once you do something about these issues, you'll
be less tempted to cope by reaching for food.

"IT'S TOO HARD!"

Managing your emotions instead of reaching for food is hard! But
so are a lot of things. Going to school, raising children, staying with
a difficult job—all of these things may take more effort than you
ever imagined. But in most cases, you do it anyway.

As an author, I often get discouraged with how hard it is to
consistently stick with my writing efforts. Natalie Goldberg, author
of *Writing Down the Bones*, teaches, "If writing was easy, everyone
would do it."

In a similar way, if losing weight was easy, there wouldn't be so
many overweight people in the world. It's not easy, yet at the same

time, it *can* be done. If you are determined to achieve your weight-loss goals, don't let the fact that it's hard get in your way.

If you're like most people, you've done many hard things and dealt with a lot of tough situations in your lifetime. Look at the challenges of carrying a pregnancy, giving birth, or caring for a sick child or an aging parent. What about changing jobs, or moving across the country?

Make a list of some of the hard challenges you've faced in your life, then remind yourself you *can* handle difficult things. Regardless of your current weight or health status, you are a strong and capable person. In fact, if you were weak or lazy, you wouldn't be reading this book.

When you're finding it hard to cope, divide your emotional challenges into small steps and tackle ones that seem easiest. Review your list of "things to do instead of eating," then choose one and focus on it until it becomes second nature. For example, instead of immediately giving in when you get a food craving, apply the "ten-minute rule" and wait ten minutes before you eat something.

Hidden Barriers

Perhaps you say you want to work on your emotional issues but never quite get around to writing your list of needs or identifying your feelings. What keeps you from applying those first steps? Certainly motivation could be part of it. But some of your roadblocks may be hidden behind years of habits or old ways of thinking.

AMBIVALENCE

Do you keep changing your mind about whether to go back on a diet or start a new exercise program? Unfortunately, being indecisive or uncertain about your goals can kill your program. And if you feel the slightest bit hesitant about working on emotional eating, you'll probably continue reaching for food instead of tackling your issues.

Ambivalence keeps you stuck. When you straddle the fence, the slightest breeze knocks you over toward the side of giving up. If you're determined to make changes in your life, kick ambivalence out the window. As you build your skills for conquering emotional eating, keep reminding yourself that you are *determined* to make this work. Then don't look back. Figure out how to achieve your goals, no matter what!

FEAR OF BEING DEPRIVED

Suppose you host a birthday party. You serve ice cream and cake to everyone, but you just drink black coffee. You want to stay on your diet, but watching everyone eat makes you feel deprived and left out. After the guests have gone home, you sneak into the kitchen and eat three pieces of birthday cake. After all, you deserve to have a little fun too, don't you?

In the past few years, numerous diet books have proclaimed "diets don't work," and the authors have coaxed us to never diet again. Theoretically, following a rigid diet plan can set up a sense of deprivation that later contributes to throwing out the rules and overeating.

This may be true for some people, but at the same time, successful weight loss does require that you set boundaries around your eating. Even if it makes you feel deprived, sometimes you'll need to turn down a piece of cake or a bowl of ice cream.

In reality, maybe deprivation isn't all that bad. In life, you deprive yourself of a lot of things because you prefer the benefits you get as a result. For example, to stay in a monogamous relationship, you deprive yourself of the pleasure of having sex with other people. When you accept a full-time job, you give up spending your days skiing or playing at the beach. But you're willing to sacrifice these things because you prefer the outcomes of staying married or getting a paycheck.

Instead of worrying about feeling deprived, define the boundaries that will keep you moving toward your goals. Like traffic laws or school-attendance policies, setting a few rules around eating keeps you from destroying your plans for staying healthy.

Maybe you've tried giving yourself "permission" to eat certain foods because that's supposed to stop cravings. Any time you feel deprived around food, look carefully at what you might "need" or "feel," not just which food you're craving.

A few years ago, I read a book that suggested giving in to food cravings rather than depriving yourself. The book said to identify the food you really want, then go ahead and eat it. Supposedly, eating what you want would stop your craving because you would no longer feel deprived of the food.

One afternoon, I decided I was craving a brownie, so I ate one. Once I finished it, I realized that it wasn't quite what I'd wanted. Instead, I was actually hungry for Oreo cookies. After eating a bunch of cookies, I sensed they weren't exactly what I wanted either. Then, I figured out that I really wanted something crunchy like M&Ms. So I got out a bag of those and finished it off. That still didn't quite do it. I don't understand why the principle of "eat what you want" doesn't seem to work for me. —Michelle

If you get a vague craving for something, look beyond your food thoughts. Before you give in to the food, do something to take care of your emotional needs first. Then if you still want the food, go ahead and eat it, but savor and appreciate it so you'll feel satisfied when you've finished eating it.

Deprivation doesn't always have to involve food. Switch it around by asking, "What does my weight deprive me of?" Are you missing out on a lot of things in life because you're overweight? Does your size keeping you from achieving some of your dreams and goals? Compared to the emotional pain of staying overweight, the minor deprivation of skipping a piece of cake starts to seem pretty unimportant.

"NO ONE TAKES CARE OF ME"

What do you do when your emotional support slips away? When you go through a divorce or other relationship changes, you can lose connections that nurtured you and made you feel emotionally safe.

Jenny knew her mother wasn't able to give her much nurturing anymore, but she couldn't figure out how to replace it.

One Saturday, I decided to visit my aging mother, who was in declining health. On the way to her home, I stopped at my favorite bakery and picked up a couple of large chocolate chip cookies. When I bit into one of those soft, chewy cookies, I was instantly overwhelmed by some of the most intense emotions I have ever felt. It was as though every part of my body suddenly filled with deep feelings of love and comfort. I don't understand why they affected me this much but the feelings were so powerful that I began to sob.
—Jenny

When Jenny thought about what happened, she realized the cookies reminded her of how her mother had always loved her and taken care of her. As her mother's health and mental ability faded, so did her nurturing role. Jenny said, "Since Mom can't take care of me anymore, I let food do it instead. I can't seem to stop eating those cookies because they replace the only way I got nurtured and loved."

Like Jenny, you may have lost a relationship that provided nurturing or comfort. Until you rebuild these missing areas of your life, you risk using food to replace them. Don't give up. Eventually the pain will heal and your ability to cope without eating will return.

IT'S TOO PAINFUL TO FACE

Grief, loss, or abandonment can bring pain almost beyond what you can bear. When her youngest son committed suicide, Frances felt like the bottom had dropped out of her world. A few weeks after the funeral, she told me, "I can't seem to get a handle on this at all. Right now, I'm just eating my way through it."

Intense emotional pain challenges all of your reserves, making it hard to not reach for food or alcohol as a way to cope. During those times, simply do everything possible to take good care of yourself. If you slip into emotional eating, work on keeping the damage as low as possible. As time passes and you rebuild your life, food will become less necessary as a way to get through the pain.

People Barriers

It seemed that every time Marilyn started a new diet plan, someone around her would have a crisis. She kept hoping her children would grow up and take care of their own lives. But they didn't. And whenever they had problems, Marilyn not only rushed in to help, she ate. As she struggled with all of her family issues, Marilyn usually ended the day by consuming a large pizza or an ice cream sundae.

A couple months ago, my daughter went through a nasty breakup with her boyfriend. For several weeks, I went over to her place every day, and when she cried, I cried with her. Then we'd get out the ice cream and eat until we both felt better.

Around this same time, my middle son lost his job. So even though I'm broke, I took over making his charge card payments to help him out. Then my oldest son called from Texas where he'd been put in jail (again) for sell-ing drugs. I was so devastated that I couldn't sleep or go to work. I just kept eating to try and not think about it. Finally, I borrowed enough money to fly down there and bail him out of jail. —Marilyn

Marilyn believed she was being a concerned and caring parent. But she also struggled with saying "no" to her own mother and to people at work. In reality, she had become so hooked into other people's lives that she had no concept of her own identity. When she tried to write down a list of her needs, she couldn't think of a single one that didn't relate to fixing someone else's problems. The only way she got her own needs met was with food.

THE PEOPLE HOOK

Marilyn become a victim of what I call the "people hook." Other people and their problems constantly hook her into feeling dis-traught, worried, and upset. At the same time, she also gets hooked into trying to fix all of their dilemmas.

The "people hook" centers on two questions:

1. How much do others influence or affect you?
2. How much do you attempt to influence or affect others?

Picture the "people hook" as three overlapping circles. The cen-ter one represents you and your efforts to take care of yourself and live your own life. The left circle symbolizes how much you are influenced or affected by others. The right circle depicts your attempts to impact other people's lives or change their behaviors.

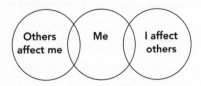

In healthy relationships, these circles overlap just a little. You care about your friends or family members, so it troubles you when they have a bad time. You also want to be helpful and kind during their struggles, so you make phone calls, meet them for coffee, and listen to their problems.

Ideally, you're able to share their sadness or show concern, but then return home and take care of yourself. When you maintain healthy boundaries, you set limits on how much you do for others. You accept that how people cope with life is their responsibility, not yours. In this picture, you have a solid identity and a clear image of your true self.

But as you get more involved in people's lives, the circles move inward toward the center. As you fret about your mother or your grown children, you end up taking care of them instead of yourself. Every new crisis pulls you further into their struggles, making you even more distraught. So when you need to escape or get relief from the stress, you reach for something to eat.

Along with worrying, you also step in and try to help whenever people around you get into trouble. Because you care about them, you try everything possible to make their lives better. However, when you become "overhooked" in other people's lives, you eventually lose sight of yourself and your own needs.

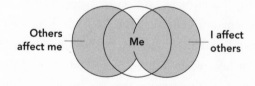

Look at the three circles now. Other people's effect on you, along with your intense efforts to help them, has overlapped the circles so far that *you* have completely disappeared. Day after day, you put your life on hold for the sake of other people's concerns.

When you become so engulfed in helping others, it's easy to let food take care of your own unmet needs.

"People hooks" aren't always your fault. For example, a car accident or a major illness can suddenly draw you into helping someone through a crisis. Even happy events like planning a wedding can temporarily engulf you. But you need to monitor how long you take care of others at your expense. Instead of giving up your own life, learn to separate other people's struggles from your own needs.

Unfortunately, when you spend a lot of your life trying to accommodate others, you seldom get what you hoped for. After all you've done for them, you might assume people will be obligated to give to you, or to love you more. But you rarely get back equal levels in return for your efforts.

Often, the people to whom you gave so much time, energy, or money will accept what you've given, then go about their own lives. Soon, you start feeling resentful because people you helped don't appreciate it and they simply take you for granted. When you don't get the gratitude or attention you hoped for, it's easy to look for it in food.

Getting "Unhooked"

Look carefully at whether "people hooks" are driving your emotional eating. If you feel like you've lost yourself as a result of taking care of others, you may have to make some hard choices about how much you help the people in your life. By giving appropriate amounts of time and energy to yourself as well as to others, you won't feel as driven to use food as a solution to your own needs.

To get out of the "people hook," you have to push the circles further apart, forcing others to manage their lives without your constant help. You also have to stop letting other people's problems devastate you. When your friends or family members call with another dilemma, determine where you can contribute and where you need to back off. Encourage people around you to take responsibility for themselves.

You can still care about people you love. Just don't let yourself disappear in the process. Pushing the circles apart will let your real self emerge from behind other people's needs. Learn to say "no" once in a while instead of trying to keep everybody happy. Remember, *your job is to love people, not fix them.*

The Perfectionism Barrier

Are you an "all-or-nothing" person? Even if you don't think it's affecting you, perfectionism can block you from reaching your goals. Most perfectionists tend to follow the same theme: *Do it right or don't do it at all.* But since they never reach the point where they can do it "right," perfectionists never start.

When you get hung up on the "right" way to do something, you lose sight of all the other possibilities. As a perfectionist, you not only apply this to yourself, you also hold a tight expectation around other people's behaviors.

LIVING IN BLACK AND WHITE

For almost every situation, you form a picture of how you think it "should" be. If you go into a bank, you expect the money to be stored in the vault, not carelessly thrown around on the counters. At a nice restaurant, you picture clean tables, attentive wait staff, and high-quality food. Think of your picture as a square, sort of a mental snapshot of what you expect.

You have expectation squares for many things in life. But sometimes you create very small mental pictures when you apply rigid

Typical expectation square

expectations to people or things around you. Unfortunately, when you hold a tight frame around a situation or a behavior, you risk being disappointed or upset because reality will never match your picture.

Rigid expectation square

Think about times you've been disappointed with something you'd hoped for. You anticipate your children will be excited when they open their holiday gifts, but instead they act hurt because they didn't get what they wanted. When you give up an entire Saturday to run errands for your grandmother, you expect her to appreciate your efforts. Instead, she complains that you should have been there last week.

You also might be holding a tight expectation square around your own behavior. Rather than set up a realistic eating plan, you design one that's rigid and overly strict. Then, if you eat a cookie that wasn't on your plan, you feel so disgusted that you give up and eat more.

If you get upset because life doesn't match your expectations, you need to widen your square and change the picture of what you consider acceptable. Apply this to your own behavior as well as to what you expect from others. Fill in the square with the new picture, then ask yourself "Could it be like this and still be okay?"

Imagine all the situations to which you could apply this concept. Suppose your child brings home a disappointing report card. What if the person in front of you at the grocery checkout has eleven items instead of ten? How about when your overworked boss snaps at you? Could you widen your expectation square to accommodate these situations? Or will you maintain a rigid set of rules for what people "should" do?

Now look at the expectations you set for yourself. What if you make one tiny slip on your diet? Does that really mean you have to go off your plan the rest of the day? If you constantly measure yourself against a rigid standard, you will seldom achieve your goal.

Rather than giving up because you set up an "all-or-nothing" expectation of yourself or others, widen your expectations to allow for more options. Work out an eating plan that allows you flexibility while still following your guidelines. Take the same approach with your exercise program or your efforts to avoid munching in response to stress. By making your pictures more flexible, you'll have a better chance of life matching them.

STEP INTO THE "GRAY"

Bob decided he was ready to start an exercise program. First he installed a lot of expensive equipment in a special carpeted area of his basement. Then he planned the ultimate workout, one that would ultimately give him the toned body of a Greek god.

His daily regimen started with twenty minutes of gentle warm-up, then moved into an intense cardiovascular workout that included half an hour on both the treadmill and an exercise bike. Then he shifted to his weight-lifting program, a meticulously planned routine that worked all of the major muscle groups in exactly the right order. His program finished with stretching and a gentle walk to cool down.

This two-hour routine was thorough and perfect for transforming him into a strong, fit individual. There was only one problem. Three months after he set up his ideal exercise program, Bob had still not done it. Not even once. You see, he could never find a two-hour block of time when he could do the whole routine. So until the day came when he could do the entire program as he'd designed it, he couldn't get himself to exercise at all.

Perfectionism usually involves "black and white thinking." You either do the whole thing (white) or you don't do it at all (black). In between these two extremes lies a gray area—a place perfectionists hate to enter. I showed Bob a graphic illustration of this principle.

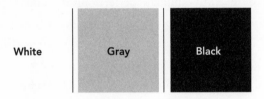

To accomplish his goals, Bob didn't need to move entirely from one extreme to the other; he just needed to put one foot into the gray area. On days when he couldn't complete the entire routine, he could simply do *part* of his workout.

Bob struggled with this concept because his brain still wanted to do the "perfect" program. But he also recognized that his rigid plan kept him from making any progress at all. So he chose to "step into the gray" instead of eliminating his entire workout.

After studying his exercise plan, Bob determined he could divide it into twenty-minute segments. He gave himself the option of doing only one segment on days when he didn't have time for the whole thing. A couple of months later, Bob reported he'd lost twenty pounds and that he was thrilled with how his workouts were going. By *changing his expectation*, he was able to do a solid twenty minutes of exercise on days he otherwise would have skipped.

If you tend to get stuck because you're thinking in this "perfectionist" way, experiment with stepping one foot into the gray. Instead of expecting yourself to "never" eat when you aren't hungry, allow for a few exceptions. Figure out how to make a small amount of progress, yet still feel successful. By letting go of your rigid rules and expectations, you'll achieve a much healthier balance in nearly every area of your life.

THINK EXCELLENCE, NOT PERFECTIONISM

You don't need to eliminate perfectionism completely. In many aspects of life, it can help you accomplish things you wouldn't otherwise achieve. Simply treat perfectionism as a wonderful gift. To maintain balance in your life, you have to decide when to use your gift and when you need to store it on a shelf. This way, you can draw on it when it matters, but other times you can choose to let it go.

You can hold high standards and strive for doing things well, but always allow yourself the option of "missing" by just a little. Set a goal of striving for "excellence" instead of perfectionism. Achieving excellence is possible with almost anything you do. By eliminating the roadblock of perfectionism, you'll have far more success in all your health behaviors, including your emotional eating.

New Thoughts and Beliefs

Henry Ford once said, "If you think you can or you think you can't, you're right." Do you ever get stuck in old "failure" messages or let negative thoughts get you down? Your thoughts have a powerful ability to affect your behaviors as well as your outcome.

If old thoughts and beliefs keep getting in the way of your progress, take a look at your vocabulary. By altering a few old messages, you'll increase your chances for success instead of failure. Here are several ideas to help you change how you talk about your efforts.

"CHOOSE TO," NOT "HAVE TO"

Think about how you respond when you say "I *have to* lose weight" or "I *have to* exercise." Most of us don't like being told we "have to" do things. In fact, that little phrase often makes you rebel and do the opposite. "I have to lose weight, but I don't feel like it, so I'm going to eat a candy bar."

In reality, you don't *have to* do anything. Suppose you say, "I have to clean my house." But in reality, some people don't. They simply leave their houses dirty. Or you argue, "I have to go to work." No, you don't. Some people live very simply or even declare bankruptcy rather than work at a job.

While it's true you don't "have to" do much of anything, you "choose" to do lots of things because you prefer the results. You consistently go to work because you like getting a paycheck. You lose weight because you want improved health and better self-esteem.

To change this barrier, eliminate "I have to" from your vocabulary. Say "I choose to. . . ." So the phrase, "I have to lose weight" becomes "I choose to lose weight." You make this choice because you want the outcome of feeling better physically or fitting into the clothes hanging in your closet.

If you say "I have to exercise" you want to avoid it even more. So change this into "I choose to walk today. I want to build my fitness level and improve my energy." Saying "I choose to" takes away the parental language that makes you feel oppressed or rebellious.

It puts *you* in charge of your own behavior, giving you more incentive to follow through with your plan.

When you feel compelled to do something, remember that you *choose* your actions. Just because your mother bakes a special cake doesn't mean you "have to" eat any of it. Unless she pushes you to the floor, shoves a piece of cake into your mouth, and makes you swallow it, you can "choose" whether or not to eat any.

Practice this technique until you feel comfortable with it. For one whole day, refer to everything you do as a *choice*. Say "I choose to get up early for my meeting" or "I choose to sit here at my desk and type this report." Notice the sense of empowerment you get from "choosing" to do activities compared with thinking you "have to" do them.

"I'll Find a Way," Not "I Can't"

When you've struggled with your weight and emotional eating for many years, you may not truly believe you can change. But don't slip into the habit of putting "I can't" in front of your goals. See if any of these comments sound familiar.

> *"I can't stay on a diet."*
> *"I can't visit my family without overeating."*
> *"I can't exercise because I don't have time."*

Saying "I can't" reinforces the belief that you're incapable of making progress. It also takes the blame off your shoulders because, after all, you "can't!" When it feels too hard to stay on your diet plan, saying "I can't" gives you a valid excuse to give up and eat.

Try this experiment. Instead of saying "I can't," say "I don't want to." Now you confess, "I don't want to stay on a diet." And you admit, "I don't want to visit my family without overeating." Stating it this way gives you a different view of your actions.

When you really do want to change your behavior, switch the words "I can't" into "I'll find a way!" Notice the difference in how you feel when you use the following statements.

"I'll find a way to stay on a diet."
"When Mom begs me to eat, I'll find a way to say no to her."
"Even though my schedule is tight, I'll find a way to exercise."

When you announce "I'll find a way," you put yourself in charge. Instead of believing you're stuck, you create new options. For example, when your mother pushes you to eat, you could tease her that she wishes you were a child again so she could "make" you do something. Once you become determined to find a way, you'll start looking for solutions instead of believing there are none.

"I USED TO... BUT NOW I'M DIFFERENT!"

Suppose you start a new diet or exercise plan. Initially, you feel excited and energized. But then a nagging voice reminds you of your past failures. You've done this before—started out strong but then lost your motivation and quit.

Secretly, you worry that this time won't be any different from the others. So when you give in to a candy bar during a bad day at work, you aren't particularly surprised. Then, since you've blown it anyway, you go ahead and eat pizza and ice cream for dinner. Soon you get frustrated because your new program isn't working and you stop completely. Just as you predicted, you gave up on your diet, like you "always" do.

Focusing on memories of past failures puts you at risk for repeating them. It's time to change your belief that things *always* go a certain way or that you *never* stay with your goals. In truth, your past struggles have no effect on your ability to succeed in the future.

So whenever you worry about repeating your old patterns, give yourself a new message. Instead of saying, "I always..." or "I never..." to describe your behaviors, replace these words with "I used to...but now I'm different!"

Maybe in the past you would stop exercising, then lose motivation to return to your program. If you fear this happening again, say to yourself, "I used to stop my exercise plan and never go back to it, but now I'm different!"

You also need to write a new ending for your statement by adding a positive step. Say "These days, I...", then complete the sentence with your new approach. For example, "If I fall off my exercise plan, I don't just give up. These days I take a long, contemplative walk and use it to get myself going again." Or you might say, "I used to eat whenever I felt stressed, but now I'm different. These days, I play relaxing music or talk to one of my friends to help manage my tension."

Any time you worry about repeating your failures, create a new belief by saying "I used to... but now I'm different." Fill in the behavior you want to change, then add a follow-up plan for how you will accomplish that goal.

———

As you move forward in your efforts to conquer emotional eating, push away the roadblocks that get in the way of your progress. Learn to recognize barriers quickly and develop ways to work around them. Keep the road cleared of anything that might prevent you from achieving your goals.

CHAPTER TEN

No More Sabotage

JUST WHEN YOU THOUGHT YOUR DIET was working great, things start to go wrong. Instead of giving you flowers on Valentine's Day, your husband hands you a large box of chocolates. Then, in the middle of your favorite TV program, your kids rip open a bag of potato chips, plunk them down on the coffee table in front of you, and ask, "Want some?"

Whatever happened to getting support for your weight-loss efforts? Does it ever seem like people are actually *trying* to make you eat? While they might not see it that way, people who wave tempting food in front of you are sabotaging your efforts to lose weight or stop your emotional eating.

As you become better at recognizing what gets in your way, you may discover that sabotage is another barrier to your success. Sabotage includes any activities or comments that undermine your efforts or prevent you from making progress. Unfortunately, these behaviors are usually the opposite of what you expect.

In fact, friends or family members you thought would be most likely to support you may act as if they want you to stay fat. Out of nowhere, they offer you treats or beg you to share a pizza or a slice of cheesecake. When you question their motives, they respond with vague answers like, "Oh, I didn't know that would bother you."

Maybe you also have times when you sabotage yourself. Once you've lost a lot of weight, do you start feeling uneasy about being thinner? Does the thought of maintaining your new weight make you panic? Maybe you aren't sure how to deal with getting more attention from members of the opposite sex. Even though you don't intend to regain, somehow you start eating more until, eventually, your weight goes back up. Once you're no longer thin, you may actually feel relieved because no one notices you anymore.

Sabotage puts you right back into the patterns of emotional eating. Maybe you want to please other people or you fear how others will act if you refuse their food. Perhaps you want to avoid failure or gain more intimacy. If you routinely become a victim of sabotage, either from yourself or other people, it's time to look at *why* you allow yourself to trip so easily.

In this chapter, you'll explore what causes sabotage along with ways to stop it from ruining your success. As with any emotional eating issue, you have to recognize the problem before you can change it. Once you realize someone is harming your progress, it's important to address it immediately instead of pretending everything's fine. If you tend to sabotage yourself, building your self-esteem and body confidence will help you manage your anxiety about losing weight or maintaining your success.

Helper or Hindrance?

Whether you're trying to lose weight, exercise more, or stop emotional eating, you want people around you to encourage you, not get in your way. Support people, or "helpers," can include your spouse or your children, other family members, friends, and coworkers. Most of the time, these people have good intentions and really want to help you accomplish your goals. But sometimes, they just don't know how to go about it.

HELPERS DON'T UNDERSTAND

Many helpers don't realize how hard it is to lose weight or stop emotional eating. So they throw out flippant comments like, "All you need to do is eat less and exercise more." They don't believe that certain foods can tempt you that much, so they ignore your requests to keep cookies or ice cream out of sight.

Some helpers go to extremes when they constantly nag you about your eating or, worse yet, when they completely ignore your efforts and never ask how you're doing. In many cases, people have learned to relate to you as an overweight person. Once you make significant changes in your lifestyle, they don't know how to act toward you.

HELPERS DON'T KNOW WHAT TO SAY

People around you may not respond to your weight-loss efforts because they aren't sure quite what to say. They're afraid that, whether they offer comments or don't say a word, you'll get mad either way. Sometimes helpers think they're supposed to watch you closely or even monitor what goes in your mouth. So when you reach for a cookie, they quickly admonish, "Should you be eating that?" When you tell them to stop being the food police, they say, "But I was only trying to help!"

Many people love to play amateur diet doctor. They question your weight-loss approach or offer pessimistic opinions like, "That's never going to work." They fret that you'll give up after a few weeks and waste all the money you've spent joining a program or purchasing special foods. If they notice you don't follow your diet perfectly, they may admonish, "Aren't you learning anything in that program?"

Some helpers have strange ideas about what will support your efforts. Stacy gained a lot of weight with her first pregnancy. Five years later, she was still struggling with an extra forty pounds.

I know my weight bothers my husband. But instead of giving me encouragement, he tries to shame me into doing something about it. He constantly teases me about my weight and makes jokes about it in front of other people. Sometimes he cuts me down by saying, "You used to look so good. What happened to your pride?"

I guess he believes that if he humiliates me enough, I'll change. But his efforts backfire because I get so hurt and angry that I stuff myself with food, making my weight go the opposite direction from what he wanted. —Stacy

Even helpers who are normally kind and sensitive may not know how to be supportive when it comes to food and eating. Many people don't know how to give praise or compliments, so they only speak up when they see you doing something wrong.

My family only pays attention to what they can see, not what they can't see. They get upset about me eating one cookie, but they don't realize that, in the past, I would eat an entire bag of cookies in an hour. —Richard

Helpers also forget that your need for support is "ongoing." Whenever she was losing weight, Betty got lots of encouragement from her coworkers. But once she reached her goal, they seemed to forget about her struggles and rarely asked how she was doing. She said, "I actually needed their support more during my first months of maintenance when I was so afraid I'd gain the weight back."

In reality, most helpers do worry about you and your struggles with eating or losing weight. They've seen you crying when you can't zip up a pair of pants that fit a year ago. They notice your fatigue or your chronic backaches. Secretly, they may feel sad at the way your struggles have affected your self-esteem or your ability to show affection. Perhaps they miss having you join them in physical activities like hiking or tennis.

But if your helpers don't express these things, you may never realize how hard they're trying. If you don't happen to notice people's efforts, you may assume they don't care. Or you might resent that they're not giving you the "right" kind of support. Sometimes your own self-esteem or emotional struggles keep you from appreciating how much your helpers are doing.

SNEAK EATING

If your helpers constantly disappoint you, it's easy to punish them for not being more supportive. When people are around, you seem to be a perfect dieter. But when no one's looking, you stuff yourself with ice cream or other snacks as a way to punish your "unhelpful" support people.

Sneak eating generally carries an attitude of "I'll show them!" Whether you're disappointed at not getting support or frustrated at how the support was given, sneak eating provides a way to get even. Out of that resentment, you end up sabotaging your own goals.

How Helpers Sabotage

When it's clear that your helpers are getting in the way of your progress, try to determine what's making them uncomfortable. Are they acting out of ignorance because they actually *don't* know how to give support? Or could they be harboring deeper feelings such as a fear of losing their power over you? Maybe they're afraid that, once you're thin, you'll leave because you won't need them anymore.

Your struggles with weight and emotional eating can easily become a battle for control. Sometimes a helper will expect perfection and become upset at the slightest hint that you've eaten something you "shouldn't" have. Some people take a rigid, military-style approach to concepts like willpower and self-discipline and have little tolerance for anything that doesn't match their rules.

In some cases, a helper may want you to stay overweight because it makes you "safe." Perhaps your spouse thinks your extra weight will make you less attractive to potential sexual partners, so you won't be likely to have an affair or stray from the relationship. Even if you did think about leaving, your helper may assume your weight would keep you from having the self-confidence to start over on your own.

Some helpers like being able to keep others dependent on them. When you're overweight, your partner can become your only source of compliments or affirmation. By convincing you that you'll never get that kind of support from anyone else, your helper makes certain you'll never leave, regardless of the abuse you endure.

INTENTIONAL SABOTAGE

Over the course of a year, Eileen worked hard at her weight-loss program and dropped nearly one hundred and fifty pounds. As her body shape changed, she began emerging from her isolation and depression. Once she gained more energy and confidence, she began to speak up for herself and her own needs.

Along with losing weight, the "new Eileen" discovered how to be more assertive and forceful in her marriage. Gradually, her husband realized he was losing his power over her. Although he appeared supportive on the surface, he made it clear that he wasn't entirely happy with her new life.

Most days, my husband acts pleasant and says things like, "I think you're doing great." But in subtle ways, he lets me know he's angry because I'm not constantly jumping to take care of him and do what he wants. I don't think he likes the changes I'm making, especially since I'm becoming more assertive.

At Christmas this year, he gave me a five-pound box of chocolates and a beautiful blouse, size 4X. However, at this point I was comfortably wearing a size 12 and the new blouse was enormous on me. After I opened my gifts, he hugged me and said he wanted the "old Eileen" back. What he really wanted was the lady who was totally dependent on him for everything, including getting compliments, attention, or affection. —Eileen

A year later, Eileen called to tell me she'd divorced her husband because he kept trying to make her fat again. Obviously, leaving a sabotaging relationship isn't the only way to cope with it. But it's critical that you recognize when you're being a victim so you can prevent the people involved from adding to your struggles.

SIGNS OF SABOTAGE

Learn to recognize when others are trying to prevent you from making changes. Here are a few signs that can indicate sabotage.

- Frequently giving you gifts of candy or high-calorie foods.
- Insisting on having chips or sweets around and in plain sight.
- Pushing you to go back to old eating habits for the sake of "togetherness."
- Begging you to go to a restaurant because they want companionship, then coercing you into eating large portions, appetizers, or desserts.
- Using food as a sign of affection or even withholding affection until you "come to your senses and eat more."

- Becoming jealous when your new body shape gets attention, particularly from members of the opposite sex.
- Saying you look ill or that you're getting "too skinny," proclaiming they "like their women/men with some meat on them."

When you suspect you're being sabotaged, evaluate whether the actions are intentional. Maybe your helpers just aren't thinking and they don't mean to be getting in the way of your progress. But if you sense that someone's clear intention is to prevent you from losing weight, you've got some work to do.

Never condone or ignore sabotage. When someone clearly demonstrates sabotaging behavior, call it for what it is. But rather than accusing the other person, seek information. Find out if your partner feels threatened by the "new you." Discuss your concerns by saying, "I don't understand your reason for tempting me with a box of chocolates."

Maybe your friends think you won't want to be around them anymore after you lose weight. They may worry about losing a "partying" buddy or the person they can always count on for sharing a pizza. To counteract this, let them know how much you value their relationships.

Reassure people that you will continue to love and appreciate them, even though you're making lots of changes in your life. Once your family or friends realize that they're still important to you, they may stop fretting about what you're trying to accomplish. If these efforts don't work, ignore their comments or avoid these people until you feel more confident about your progress.

SIDESTEPPING SABOTAGE

Has this ever happened to you? You mention to someone that you're trying to lose weight, and right away, that person pushes you to eat something. Some people take the word "diet" as a personal challenge to see whether they can make you fall off the wagon. They beg you to "have a few chips" or meet them at a new buffet-style restaurant. When you protest, they push you harder.

To defeat this type of sabotage, you have to stay in charge of your own behavior. The best way to win the "I can make you eat" game is to not even play. Rather than eat just to get people off your back, use subtle methods to get them to stop.

I've already eaten. Convince others you don't need any food. Tell them you've already eaten and right now are quite full. Or let them know that you're planning to eat somewhere else later. For example, you might beg off by saying, "I'd better not eat anything because Mom is expecting me and she's cooking a big meal." If people believe your food needs are taken care of, they'll be less likely to push you to eat.

You can also blame your weight-loss program for why you don't want to eat. When someone pressures you about your food decisions, you can escape by saying, "The leader of my program suggests we avoid talking about our dieting efforts because it makes us think about food. Do you mind if we change the subject?"

Not right now. Another way to get rid of food pushers is to assure them you will eat later. When someone offers you food, say "Not just yet; I'm going to wait a little while." This magic phrase convinces people you will eat eventually, so they leave you alone.

Whenever they return and offer you food again, simply repeat the phrase or some variation of it. You might say, "Thanks, but I'll still wait a bit" or "Not right now, but maybe later."

You can use these lines repeatedly at gatherings and most people will never realize you didn't eat during the event. Saying "not right now" provides a gracious way to manage the discomfort of feeling pushed to eat when you don't want food.

Training Your Helpers

You may need to teach your helpers how to give you the kind of support that works for you. Most people want to encourage you— they just need guidance on how to be an effective support person.

INCREASE THEIR AWARENESS

Sit down with your helpers and explain *why* you are working so hard to stop emotional eating or stay on your diet plan. Share your goals and your plans for achieving them. Describe your specific intentions, such as eating dessert only once a week, limiting alcoholic drinks, or ordering salads with the dressing on the side.

Remind your helpers that what they see is only a small part of your plan. Then tell them about what they *can't* see—how you've curbed your emotional eating responses, stopped your McDonald's run on the way home from work, and eliminated your extra snacks.

ASK FOR HELP

Give clear instructions on the type of help you want. Instead of saying, "Please help me lose weight" or "Be nicer to me," clarify what you mean. Do you want your family members to eat their snacks in another room rather than in front of you? Then let them know.

With specific requests, start by saying, "It will help me if...", followed by what you want people to do. For example, you might say, "It will help me not to have chips in the house right now. Would you be willing to eat them with your lunch at work instead of bringing them home?"

When you start digging through the cupboards, perhaps you'd like your helper to ask whether you're feeling "hungry" or you're just having a "desire to eat." Maybe you'd love to hear your partner say, "I notice you seem to be struggling with your eating today. Are you feeling or needing anything particular?"

Let your helpers know how you want them to handle social situations. Do you enjoy being praised or having other people affirm your progress? Or would you prefer they not say anything about your looks or your weight for a while? Let your helpers know which responses feel good compared to the ones that make you uncomfortable.

Feel free to let people know what you *don't want*. If it bothers you to be teased or have your weight discussed in front of your friends, ask your helpers not to do that. Be specific about which phrases particularly set you off. Let people know you hate being called nicknames like "Tubs" or having someone ask, "Is that on your diet?"

Make a list of behaviors you want your helpers to avoid, like snatching your plate, giving lectures, or admonishing, "You're not supposed to be eating that." As you make progress, be sure to let your helpers know if your needs have changed and you don't need their support as much.

Explain What You Want

Use this next exercise to tell your helpers what you want from them in specific situations. Pick out the answers that fit best for you, then read the statements aloud to your family members or friends. This gives your helpers a clear message about what you *do* find useful as well as the responses you *don't* want to hear. Consider posting the list on the refrigerator or in some other location where people can remind themselves of what you said.

Appreciate Good Helpers

When people give you solid, helpful support, let them know you appreciate it. Be willing to share the stories about your progress, particularly in areas other than the changes on the scale. Show your friends the exercises in this book and ask them to help you practice skills like identifying your needs or expressing your feelings.

Remind helpers that you are involved in a lifelong project, not one that will be finished by the summer or the holidays. Ask people to support you in achieving goals that are realistic, not push you

What I Want from You

1. If you see me eating something that's not on my plan:

___ Ask me if I've had a bad day.

___ Ignore it entirely.

___ Give me a hug.

___ Other _____.

2. When I'm making noticeable progress, i.e., losing weight:

___ Compliment me on how I look.

___ Praise me in front of others.

___ Don't comment on my progress in front of others.

___ Give me non-food gifts or rewards.

___ Other _____.

3. When I'm struggling or gaining weight:

___ Tell me you notice and really care about my struggle.

___ Ignore it entirely.

___ Hug me and show me extra affection.

___ Ask me how you can help.

toward becoming a body builder or a model. Let them know you want to be accepted as you are, even with your imperfections.

Always accept compliments and praise graciously. Be careful not to discount people's comments because of your own frustrations. For example, if someone remarks that you look great since you've

___ Other _____.

4. When I'm making progress you can't see (like improving my self-esteem):

___ Ask me how my efforts are going.

___ Compliment me on how I look.

___ Ignore my efforts and changes.

___ Give me non-food gifts or rewards.

___ Other _____.

5. When I've maintained my weight (even though I may still want to lose):

___ Tell me you're proud of my current efforts.

___ Ignore the subject entirely.

___ Ask me if I'm struggling or feeling discouraged.

___ Compliment me on my looks and my efforts.

___ Other _____.

What you are welcome to say or do:_____
_____.

What I'd prefer you not say or do: _____
_____.

lost weight, don't minimize their words by saying, "Yes, but I still have such a long way to go." This can make them think their support doesn't mean a thing to you. Thank them and say, "You can't imagine how much it helps me to hear you say those things. Thank you!"

Avoid asking "set up" questions that helpers can't answer honestly. Here are some examples.

• Does this dress make me look fat?
• Can you tell if I've lost any weight?
• Does my fat stomach bother you?

Helpers hate these questions! They know that either you'll get upset with their answers or you'll accuse them of not telling the truth. When you feel insecure or struggle with your self-esteem, work on overcoming these issues instead of punishing your helpers.

RECOGNIZE BAD HELPERS

Occasionally, you'll encounter people who don't know how to be good helpers but feel it is their duty to give you advice. It's not unusual to hear negative, degrading comments from everyone from your family doctor to people you don't even know.

When someone says hurtful or insensitive things, deflect the comments rather than take them personally. You might say, "I need your help, not your scolding." Or you might simply agree by responding, "You may be right," then talking about something else.

If someone criticizes the way you're eating or the fact you aren't losing weight, thank them for being concerned. Then say, "I'm actually working on a lot of issues in my life right now and my weight is only one of them."

No one can *make* someone else lose weight or stop emotional eating. If your helpers get impatient during times when you're struggling, offer them guidance on how to give you support when you aren't doing well. Let them know it's not their fault—they aren't responsible for you making changes in your life. Appreciate their concern by saying, "It's so nice to know that, when I'm ready to work on this, you'll be here for me."

Self-Sabotage

Other people can certainly make it difficult to change your behaviors. But what about the times you sabotage yourself? Have you ever lost weight, then almost intentionally eaten enough to make sure you would gain it right back?

What about times you plan to do self-care things (such as completing the exercises in this book), but never follow through? Do you keep putting off your actions until "some day" when you'll feel more like doing it?

Sometimes *not* taking action is legitimate. If you're too busy or too stressed to start something new, it makes sense to wait a while. But you may be avoiding the very steps you know will make your life different. Is it possible you don't want to change? If you keep making excuses for not taking action, maybe you have a hidden desire to keep things the same.

Perhaps you hold yourself to high standards and expect perfection from yourself. So when you slip up, you decide to punish yourself for not being perfect. Even though your stomach is bloated and you feel terrible, you force yourself to eat more and increase your misery.

Although these behaviors may not seem like self-sabotage, they certainly don't build your motivation. If you consistently prevent yourself from reaching your goals, start looking at why you resist making progress.

WEIGHT AS PROTECTION

If you frequently sabotage yourself, you may actually *need* to stay overweight or continue emotional eating. Perhaps losing weight is too scary or you don't feel confident or comfortable as a thin person. If you've been a victim of rape, incest, or other abusive behavior, your weight may be helping you feel safe. Subconsciously, you may believe that if you lose weight, something bad will happen.

At age 23, Janice was raped inside a friend's college dorm room. Through several years of counseling and the support of her family and friends, she gradually recovered from the trauma. But during this time, she discovered food gave her a lot of comfort and nurturing. By graduation, she'd gained seventy pounds.

Over the next ten years, Janice tried many times to lose her extra weight, but whenever she got within twenty-five or thirty pounds of her goal, she started to feel anxious and uneasy. Occasionally she fought nightmares or was afraid even in broad daylight. To compensate for her anxiety, Janice would eat more, soon gaining back much of the weight she'd lost.

Finally Janice recognized that whenever she got close to what she weighed at the time of the rape, she would feel vulnerable, unsafe, and fearful that it could happen again. Without being aware of it, she would eat until her weight went back up to a point where she felt emotionally safe and protected from being attacked.

To overcome sabotaging herself, Janice had to create a belief that she *could* be safe, regardless of her weight. She enrolled in a self-defense class and learned karate and kickboxing. After taking a course in assertiveness, she began counseling employees on sexual harassment issues. Once she learned how to create her own sense of emotional and physical safety, she was able to reach her goals and maintain them without difficulty.

AVOIDING INTIMACY

Your size can also protect you from getting involved in relationships or facing the prospect of physical intimacy. If you've been a victim of abuse or you feel extremely self-conscious about your body, you may not want to deal with getting close to someone.

As long as you stay overweight, people aren't likely to approach you about having sex or an intimate relationship. You can function in your own world, choosing whether to become involved with others or simply avoid them.

You may not experience these fears until you've lost a lot of weight. As you start looking more attractive, people are more likely to give you approval and sexual attention. If you don't trust your ability to handle this added attention, you may let your diet slip. Before you know it, you've gained back enough weight so that you no longer get noticed.

Some women are even afraid that once they open themselves up to sexual experiences, they will lose control in the same way they do with food. Instead of being able to enjoy a healthy sexual relationship, these women are terrified that they'll become promiscuous. Rather than learn how to build stronger confidence in their ability to manage intimacy and closeness, they simply gain back enough weight to eliminate the risk of sexual involvement.

If you've been living without intimate relationships for a long time, staying fat provides a way to keep your sexual feelings dormant. Norma is a 38-year-old overweight accountant who has been divorced for several years. She has a good job, several close friends, and a cozy house that she shares with her two cats.

Most of the time, Norma feels comfortable with her life and rarely thinks about dating or sexual relationships. However, when she loses weight, she starts getting back in touch with her body.

I can go for years without thinking about sex, but once I lose weight, all of that changes. I start noticing men a lot more and then I also feel more lonely and isolated. Sometimes, I actually start missing sex. But I don't really want to start dating or looking for a serious relationship, so having those sexual thoughts just frustrates me. Dealing with all of these things feels like too much work—it's a lot easier to just skip it. So I gain back the weight and soon all of those feelings go away. —Norma

HOW YOUR WEIGHT SPEAKS

Being overweight can make you feel sturdy and powerful. Unlike a petite person, your size alone communicates the message "Don't mess with me!" If you've been able to intimidate people because of your size, you may be afraid that losing weight will take away that power.

Staying overweight also lets you hide from people and avoid getting involved in many aspects of life. You avoid the embarrassment of gaining weight back because you never lose it to begin with. Maybe you're convinced you can't change your life until you lose weight. But in reality, you may not be able to lose weight until you change your life!

Brenda admitted she couldn't face the work involved with dieting or even maintaining a lower weight. She said, "Being thin is like getting pregnant. You not only have to deal with this tiny baby, you have to raise it for the next twenty years. If I lose weight, I'll have to constantly monitor myself in order to maintain it. I just don't have the energy or motivation to do that."

WEIGHT AS PUNISHMENT

Two years ago, Connie's husband had an affair. After it ended, he begged for forgiveness and promised he'd never stray again. Connie accepted his apology and his efforts to rebuild their relationship.

Things went well except for one minor problem—Connie's weight.

When she had first gained a few pounds, Connie noticed her husband was hurt, because he detests heavy women. So she gained a little more. In some ways, she feels like it's payback time. She knows her husband is committed to staying with her, but by not trying to lose weight, she can keep punishing him for the affair.

Weight can also be used to punish *yourself*. If you don't believe you deserve to be thin or happy, staying overweight guarantees these things will remain out of your reach. Your weight becomes a self-limiting curse. Because you can only shop in stores that carry extra-large sizes, you can't wear attractive clothes. You can't even consider participating in sports like hiking or tennis. So staying overweight becomes your punishment for emotional eating.

Letting Go of Your Past

When you have painful memories about certain life events, you can become obsessed with figuring out how to heal from them. If you don't believe you can make progress in other areas until you "get over" these things, you may never achieve your weight-loss goals or overcome your emotional eating.

CRAP IN THE BACKYARD

Instead of dwelling on your past, learn how to acknowledge it, then let it go. Here's a simple exercise to help you accomplish this. Picture yourself living in a small house with a fenced backyard. When you step out into that yard, you realize that all you see is *crap*. The whole backyard is filled with bad things that have happened in your life—physical or sexual abuse, emotional beatings, divorce, loss, disappointment.

In attempting to work through these issues, you may have already spent years in this backyard. You've dug up every inch of that crap, looked it over, and studied parts of it closely. Perhaps you've rearranged it, sorted it, or tried to bury it deeper. But despite all your efforts, the fact remains that what's out there is still crap. No matter what you do, you can't get rid of those bad things. They remain a part of your life and, like it or not, they'll always stink.

During the years of working in that yard, you may have picked up some insights or learned some things about yourself. But at some point, you need to complete the learning and start to move on. When the time is right, make a clear decision to leave the crap behind.

Close the back door tightly, turn around, and walk the other direction until you go out the front door. Take a deep breath, enjoy the sunshine, then start planting flowers. In your front yard, cultivate a wide variety of beautiful things—kindness, patience, joy, excitement, and talent.

Digging around in crap every day doesn't make you better. Of course, the backyard will always stay hidden behind the house. If you need to, every once in a while go look into the yard and say, "Yes, that's a lot of crap!" Then leave it there, close the door, and go back to your flowers.

Many current theories hold that you don't have to remember all of your past in order to get better. Even with a history of traumatic childhood events, you don't have to pull apart every detail before you can recover. Rather than holding on to your anger or grief or bitterness, decide which specific areas you need to do additional work in. Then leave the rest dormant in the backyard and focus on moving forward in your life.

Overcoming Sabotage

The road to overcoming emotional eating gets smoother once you get past the behaviors that harm your progress. Keep watching for any signs of sabotage, from others as well as from yourself. If you recognize sabotaging behavior, deflect it—don't allow it to stop your efforts.

Whenever you sabotage yourself, try to identify what's behind your actions. If your struggles relate to a need to feel safe, learn how to protect yourself in other ways. Do activities that will help you believe that you're safe at a lower weight. Work on your self-esteem and cultivate confidence that you can be strong and capable, no matter what your size.

Build a team of helpers and support people, then train them to provide the kind of help you need. At the same time, become your own best friend and learn how to kick away sabotaging thoughts before they get a chance to do harm.

CHAPTER ELEVEN
What Will I Do?

ALL THE UNDERSTANDING IN THE world won't help much unless you *do* something with what you know. Without a solid plan for implementing what you've learned, this book will sit on the shelf with all the other self-help guides you've read but never used. So now it's time to create an action plan that will launch you out of your chair and into making progress.

Action plans don't have to be complicated. Just take a few steps toward altering your behaviors, then follow those changes with a few more. Soon you will have defined a new path, one that leads you to coping successfully with life's challenges *without* reaching for food.

While this book focuses primarily on conquering emotional eating, most of the techniques also apply to exercise, managing stress, and maintaining balance in your life. If you tend to procrastinate with projects like writing a report or cleaning the house, you can use these tools to help you leap into action. Don't wait until you've read this book through to the end before getting started. As you move through this chapter, take steps *now* toward renewing your life.

Return to What Works

The secret to your future may lie in your past. Think back to previous times when you've accomplished goals like losing weight or exercising regularly. What helped you stick with your program? How did you keep yourself on track, even through difficult times?

Use the following questions to remember what helped you before:

- What was I doing that made my efforts successful?
- Which factors are the same today as back then?
- Which ones are different?
- What helped me stay on target when I was struggling?
- What didn't work? What made me lose focus or quit?

Look at similar goals you want to accomplish now. Can you recall any techniques or creative ideas that would work for you again? Even one small solution from the past can boost your progress with your current plan.

What about periods when you managed your emotions without using food to cope? How were you different at that time? Were you less stressed? Not as angry? More comfortable with your body?

Even if your life has changed, you can still draw on what worked for you in the past. Simply pull your best strategies off the shelf and actively pursue them again. Maybe you laid your exercise clothes out at night or kept a water bottle in the refrigerator so you could grab it easily before you started your walk. Recall the tiniest details that helped you stick with your efforts, then use those as a foundation for your current plan.

Here are some of the skills my clients recalled from their past successes.

- *I would mentally shout "NO!" whenever I was tempted to eat desserts or sweets.*
- *I talked about my feelings a lot more.*
- *Instead of taking a coffee break, I did deep-breathing exercises to manage my stress.*
- *I went dancing every week. It always helped me work off my frustration.*
- *I took out my anger on the weeds in my garden.*
- *I attended a weight-loss support group every week.*

Is your life more difficult than it was a few years ago? A physical injury, a job change, or a divorce can all change the way you cope with life. But don't let your present circumstances keep you from making action plans. Instead of getting stuck on what you *can't* do, figure out what you *can* salvage from your past. Some of the self-talk phrases or mental images that helped you before might work again.

Setting Up for Success

When you draw up your action plans, be sure they match *you* and *your* current situation, not someone else's. Creating a grandiose plan won't guarantee you'll follow through with it. For example, running a marathon or climbing a mountain might intrigue you. But you've never gone running or taken a hike in your life. So, right now, maybe you just need to buy new socks so your walking shoes won't hurt your feet.

Action plans also need to fit with your personal goals and values. If you tend to be kind and soft-spoken, you don't need to become loud and mean to express your feelings. You can learn how to speak about your emotions in ways that match your personality.

BE REALISTIC

Suppose you start a new workout program with the goal of getting "back in shape." Because you're determined to make progress quickly, you push yourself hard. But after a few days, your muscles hurt, you feel exhausted, and you can't bring yourself to endure that level of punishment again. So you stop your exercise plan and never return to it.

If your program is so intense that you give up before you've barely started, then your action plan probably wasn't realistic. Start with setting goals you *know* you can accomplish. If taking a ten-minute walk during your lunch break seems more feasible than a thirty-minute run after work, go with the lunchtime walk.

Changing your behavior won't always feel comfortable or easy. But at the same time, if you hate everything on your action plan, you won't stay with it for long. So even when you stretch your comfort zone, look for ways to feel physically and emotionally safe.

For example, if you can't force yourself into a leotard in order to attend an exercise class, you might decide to use workout videos at home. If talking about your emotions feels too uncomfortable, record them in a journal until you build confidence in expressing them out loud. Whenever you tackle an especially challenging goal, you can make it more tolerable by integrating a little pleasure or comfort.

A few years ago, I bought a new bicycle thinking it would help me get more exercise. The first few times I rode it, I was miserable. My back hurt, my crotch got sore, and I certainly didn't have much fun. So I went back to the sporting goods store and asked how to make my bike more comfortable. I left the shop with a new set of handlebars that positioned my body more upright and a "gel" bike seat that provided cushioning in the places I needed it. Those simple changes transformed bike riding into one of my favorite activities.

Build a Picture

To aim for a goal, you need to know what it looks like. Vague goals produce poor results, so when you set up action plans, make them as specific as you can. Start by building a photo-sharp vision of the outcome you want to achieve.

If you're a "visual" person, you probably won't have much trouble creating a clear picture of your goals. However, some people are more inclined to "hear" or "feel" mental images as opposed to seeing them. If you tend not to "see" things easily, build a goal picture using the mental style that works best for you.

See It, Hear It, Feel It

See positive images. Always use strong, positive images to enhance your motivation. If you have a photo of yourself at a healthy weight, tape it on your mirror or refrigerator. Surround yourself with helpful symbols and visual reminders. Pick out a favorite "thin" clothing outfit and hang it where you can see it every day. Use it to remind yourself why you're working so hard to reach your goals.

Don't try to inspire your actions by using a negative image, such as taping a picture of a fat pig on the refrigerator door. Your brain can't distinguish between a positive image and a negative one, and it will try to help you match the pictures in front of it. So when it sees a pig every day, your brain will think you want to be one. Rather than setting yourself up for failure, use positive images to provide your inspiration.

Hear your progress. If you learn best by "listening," read your goals and affirmations out loud. Hearing the words, "I now weigh one hundred and forty pounds" or "I'm feeling great" will strengthen your belief that you can make these things happen.

You can also make a tape or CD recording of your own voice describing your success. Every morning while you prepare for the day, play your recording and let your own words inspire your actions.

Feel your success. If you tend to "feel" things, concentrate on how your body will feel when you reach the outcome you want. Picture yourself moving easily through a row of theater seats. Imagine your toned muscles lifting a child or pulling weeds from your garden. If you struggle with tension, recall the sense of deep relaxation that follows a massage.

For years, Dan had maintained his weight and fitness level by running every day. Then a knee injury and other problems caused him to give up his exercise program. Two years and forty pounds later, he attempted to return to his workouts. When he tried to visualize a positive outcome, he couldn't "see" how his body would look at a healthy weight. But he easily remembered how it "felt." During the years he was exercising consistently, he would imagine himself being like a deer, gracefully leaping over rocks and fences as he ran.

Dan used his "feeling" memory to inspire his current exercise program. He recalled the ease of his breathing, the strength of his legs, and his clear thinking and mental focus. By drawing on the memory of how he felt in the past, Dan got his running program to work again.

REVERSE NEW YEAR'S RESOLUTION

Usually we make New Year's Resolutions on January 1st, then spend the year trying to make them happen. But instead of waiting until next year to set new resolutions, I want you to pretend you've already achieved the goals you set for yourself. In this exercise, you assume you've conquered your emotional eating habits, lost weight, or built up to a strong fitness level. Imagine yourself looking and feeling exactly the way you want.

Mentally fast-forward to one year from now. Picture—in detail—how you want to look, feel, and live, now that you've met the goals you set today. Be realistic as you create your list, but don't be afraid to dream big. Set your sights on accomplishing each one of these goals over the next twelve months.

In your notebook or on a piece of paper, write "The date now is _____, and here's what I've accomplished." Then fill in the blank with today's month and day exactly one year from now. For each of the statements, write an answer based on what you'd like to see happen in your life.

Reverse New Year's Resolution

The date is _____ (exactly one year from today)
Here's what I've accomplished

I now weigh: _____
(the weight you desire and believe is realistic one year from now)

My body feels: _____
(*strong, healthy, slender, thinner, toned, flat, etc.*)

I'm exercising by: _____
(*walking, biking, three to four times per week*)

I'm pleased with: _____
(*expressing emotions, self-nurturing, body changes, new attitude*)

I've learned: _____
(*how to cope with stress, ways to manage emotional eating, etc.*)

One sentence that describes my life today (Dream big on this one!):
_____
_____

_____

After you complete your statements, read your resolutions out loud. How do you feel as you hear yourself describing your future? Does it sound possible? Wonderful? Scary? Are you skeptical this outcome will ever happen?

Very likely, you will experience all of these responses. Of course, you have work to do between now and next year, but the picture you've just created *can* come true. Keep your Reverse New Year's Resolution where you can read it every day. Each time you review those words, you reinforce your potential to make them a reality.

Julie wanted to lose fifty pounds. Lately, she'd been allowing her emotions to ruin her diet plan. She had also stopped exercising and couldn't seem to get started again. See how Julie created her Reverse New Year's Resolution, below.

Julie's Reverse New Year's Resolution

**The date is: One year from now
Here's what I've accomplished**

I now weigh: One hundred and forty pounds.

My body feels: Light, strong and toned.

I'm exercising by: Walking twenty minutes a day, five or six days a week.

I'm pleased with: The way I've learned to nurture myself without using food to do it. My ability to express my feelings to my husband and kids.

I've learned: I don't need to eat every time I want to feel better. Now I reach for my "instead" list and use other ways to improve my day.

My life today: I'm thrilled that I'm maintaining my goal weight, managing my emotions in ways that don't involve food, and feeling a lot more at peace in my life.

Julie was amazed at how motivated she felt after reading her resolution. Seeing the goals as if she'd already met them inspired her to get back on track. Now she writes a Reverse New Year's Resolution at least once a year. Holding a vision of how she will be the next year gives her great motivation to push forward with her goals.

Create an Action Plan

Once you set your goals, you need a practical system to help you reach them. Start by defining your "intention" and specifying *exactly* what you want to accomplish. You can state an intention as either an outcome or an action. Make your goals measurable so you can assess whether or not you did them. For example, if you set the intention of taking a walk today, by evening you can report whether you took the walk or not.

WHAT WILL IT TAKE?

Choose a goal or activity you want to accomplish, write it down, then ask, "What will it take to make this happen?" Come up with a specific action to follow through with your intention. Label your answer "What will it take?" (As a shortcut, you can use "WWT" to abbreviate the phrase.)

Each time you define an action step, your answer becomes your new intention. That means you have to decide on an action step for this new goal. For example, if your intention is to lose twenty pounds, you might decide to go back on a diet plan you've used in the past. With this as your intention, you now have to determine a specific action to achieve that goal, like getting the menus and instructions out of a storage box so you can start using the diet.

As you create your plans, keep asking, "What will it take?" over and over, each time moving closer toward an action you can't escape, no matter what. Label your final action step as a "NOW" goal. Then get up from your chair and *do* it.

Suppose you decide to walk during your lunch break at work, but you keep forgetting to bring your walking shoes. The example below shows how you can use the "What will it take?" principle to achieve your goal. Remember that each WWT answer becomes your next intention.

Think about goals that you never make progress with, even though you've had them for years. Maybe you keep saying you want to lose weight or learn yoga. If you always "say" you want to accomplish something, but never do it, look for the holes in your system.

Start by evaluating your goal. Is it really something you want to do? Do you need more time or money to make it happen? Would it help to simplify your goal or state it a different way? Maybe you need to alter your plan to make it more palatable. Doing a thirty-minute

What Will It Take?

What is my intention? To walk every day at lunchtime.

WWT? Have my gym shoes at my desk.

What is my intention? Bring gym shoes to work.

WWT? Put them in the car when I get home this evening.

What is my intention? Put gym shoes in car this evening.

WWT? Stick a note on my briefcase to remind myself.

What is my intention? Write a note to remind myself.

WWT? Do it right now.

run might seem like a wonderful goal, but if you haven't been exercising for several years, then initially you may need to set an intention of walking for ten minutes or three city blocks.

In addition, make your intentions *specific* and *measurable*. If you just say you want to "lose weight," how will you know when you've reached your goal? Be specific: State your intention as reaching a certain number on the scale or fitting into a specific clothing size.

If you set a reasonable intention but still don't follow through with it, you may have left too many gaps in your action plan. Don't allow yourself to get out of the job. Keep digging deeper into "What will it take?" until you find an action you can't escape. Designate this final step as a NOW goal, then complete the task immediately.

Working Your Plan

Setting intentions works for everything from tiny goals like taking a walk to big plans like losing a hundred pounds or participating in a race. To accomplish a major action plan, break your goals down into smaller intentions that you can accomplish easily.

Remember Julie's New Year's Resolution to lose fifty pounds? See how she developed her action plan on page 209. In her case, she didn't restate each answer as a new intention, but she still used the "What will it take?" (WWT?) principle to keep searching for actions she could do right away.

Moving Forward

Remember, action leads to action. Build momentum by stepping from one NOW goal to the next on your list. Work through your action plan until you've passed the crisis point and know you can resist the temptation to give in to food.

Julie's Plan
What is my intention?

Stay on a solid diet and exercise program until I weigh one hundred and forty pounds, then follow a healthy maintenance plan.

1. What is my intention? Choose a diet plan for this project.

WWT? Go back to the physician-based program I used before.
WWT? Call the doctor's office for current information on program times.
WWT? Find the phone number and call during lunch.
WWT? Get out the phone book and write the number down.
WWT? Get up from my desk and get the phone book off the shelf.

2. What is my intention? Set up an exercise program.

WWT? Renew my membership at the health club; work with a personal trainer.
WWT? Stop at the club and sign up for a meeting with a trainer.
WWT? Plan it into my schedule for sometime this week.
WWT? Pull out my schedule book, write it into a day that works.
WWT? Do it now!

3. Manage emotional eating patterns.

WWT? Figure out a way to stop using food to manage my stress.
WWT? Come up with a better way to relax after work.
WWT? Use a journal to write out my feelings and thoughts related to the day.
WWT? Go to the bookstore on Saturday to buy a new journal.
WWT? Tell the kids they can go with me and listen to "story hour."

When your intentions center on changing your emotional eating patterns, you can still focus on NOW goals. Simply match them to what you need and feel, setting up actions that prevent you from reaching for food.

Whenever you need an instant solution to a food temptation, ask yourself whether you need to calm down, build your energy, or just feel nurtured. Then pick the need that feels strongest and tackle that one first. Just doing *something* often strengthens your ability to follow through with other action plans on your list

Don't lose sight of the wonderful things you've learned about how to handle your emotional needs. If you drift back into "I know what to do, I just don't do it," pull out your action plans and remind yourself of what you know.

Once a month or so, review the tools you've learned. Reread them, turn them over in your mind, and remember how it feels to use them. Each day that you stand strong against emotional eating, you also move forward in your efforts to successfully manage your weight.

CHAPTER TWELVE

Unstuck and Motivated

WHEN YOU'RE BATTLING EMOTIONAL eating, motivation affects everything! Motivation provides the *power* behind all of your action plans and helps you follow through with your good intentions. Staying motivated doesn't mean you have to be excited and energized all the time. You just have to know how to crank yourself back up when you need a boost.

Motivation tends to be mysterious and elusive. You don't usually know exactly how you got it started. And when it leaves, you have no idea where it went or how to get it back. When your motivation is strong, you may not even realize it or give it much thought. But once it slips away, you certainly know how it feels to not have it.

So what is motivation? Ironically, defining motivation is easier if you look at what it is *not*. For most people, having no motivation is feeling tired, frustrated, stuck, discouraged, or even hopeless. Although you *say* you want to exercise or eat healthier, you don't do anything about it. Staying on the couch is a lot easier than riding your exercise bike. And the fast-food restaurant down the street always looks more appealing than recipes in your low-fat cookbook.

Solid motivation is just the opposite. When your motivation is high, you feel energized, driven, focused, and determined. Nothing gets in your way and you sail through your day, pleased with yourself and your actions. Motivation provides the *push* that makes you do what needs to get done.

Once you're motivated, you can do anything, even if you hate it. You jump into action and clean the house, exercise, or write a letter to a friend. None of this seems like a problem; you just *do* it. If only you could figure out how to make that energy stick around!

But before you know it, something sneaks in and zaps your motivation away. Perhaps you get a bad cold or have a family crisis. Or you get sidetracked because you move to a different home, change jobs, or start dating someone new. Before long, your enthusiasm slips away and you're right back where you started. The house gets dirty again, your weight creeps back up, and your exercise bike becomes a clothes rack.

When Motivation Leaves

Eric really wants to stay consistent with his exercise plan. When his motivation is strong, he gets up early every day and heads out for a long run. Not even bad weather, fatigue, or work pressures stop him from following his daily routine. But every once in a while, he goes through periods when he loses motivation. Then he fights what he calls the "major gap between Sunday-night resolve and Monday-morning reality."

I'm so determined the night before. But then the alarm rings while it's still dark outside and my body feels like there's a truck parked on top of it. I recite affirmations, I use positive self-talk, and I promise myself rewards.

But nothing gets me out from under those covers. I shut off the stupid alarm and turn over for another hour of sleep.—Eric

Motivation takes energy. Any time you feel exhausted, overwhelmed, or highly stressed, you struggle to get yourself going. You know exercise would make you feel better, you just can't bring yourself to do it. Somehow, you need to learn how to push yourself out the door for a walk instead of sinking into the recliner.

INTERESTED OR COMMITTED?

How committed are you to achieving your goals? If you aren't sure, take a look at the difference between the words *interested* and *committed*.

If you're only "interested" in something, you tend to get distracted easily and might change your mind about whether it's important. When something better comes along, you go off in a new direction. For example, maybe you were interested in losing weight, but then someone brought doughnuts to the office, so you decided to quit being on a diet.

"Interested" people tend to fall into "if only" thinking. "If only I had more time (more money, a new job, a supportive spouse), I'd be a lot more motivated." When you're just "interested," you let your feelings determine your actions. As long as you feel like it, you stay on your diet or exercise plan. But if you get tired or depressed, you let it all go.

On the other hand, being "committed" means you follow through with your goals, *no matter what*. Instead of blaming circumstances for your failures, you stay with your efforts despite not having things like enough money or time or supportive people. Because you focus on actions, not feelings, you follow your diet or exercise plan even when you don't feel like it.

Think carefully about how you feel right now: Are you "committed" to your goals or just "interested" in reaching them? To build strong motivation, you have to improve your level of commitment.

Motivation Is a Choice

What can you do when you lose your motivation and don't know how to get it back? Motivation doesn't drop out of the sky or suddenly reappear after an absence. You can't open your junk drawer and exclaim, "Look! I just found my motivation!" Instead, the drive and energy that keeps you on track originates inside of you.

Motivation is a *choice*. You create it yourself—through your thoughts, your self-talk, and your attitudes. Even when you don't have a shred of energy, you can still access your motivation if you want to. You just have to get up out of your chair and *make* it happen. Here are some ideas for creating lasting motivation.

SET YOUR INTENTIONS

Motivation needs an outcome. Abstract goals like "I want to lose weight" don't generate lasting resolve. You have to set intentions that are *specific* and *measurable*. For example, you might set an intention like "I want to weigh one hundred and forty pounds by September" or "I want to run a three-mile race without having to slow down to a walk." Having specific goals that you can visualize now and measure once they're completed will motivate you much more than a vague "I'll try this and see how it goes."

When you work on major changes, divide your overall goal into smaller mini-goals, rather than tackle it all at once. Sherry was totally overwhelmed with the prospect of having to lose one hundred and fifty pounds. So she decided to stay on her diet program until she had lost twenty-five pounds, then reevaluate her plan.

When she reached that goal, she thought carefully about her efforts, then decided to lose another twenty-five pounds.

Sherry did this six times during her program, always evaluating her plans at the end of each twenty-five-pound loss. In the beginning, she couldn't imagine reaching her weight-loss goal, but by the end of the year, she'd lost the entire one hundred and fifty pounds.

TAKE SMALL STEPS

Any time you aim for perfection or set unrealistic standards, motivation won't stick around for long. Particularly with exercise, suddenly deciding "I've got to do *something*" can make you overzealous. But if you overdo on your workout, you get stiff and sore, you hate how you feel, and you just quit. When you give up, you blame your failure on lack of motivation instead of unrealistic expectations.

At Judy's weight-loss program, the participants always set an exercise goal for the following week. But Judy refused to participate in that part of the class. She said, "I hate exercise and I just don't want to do it." The other members supported her decision and encouraged her to keep attending the group anyway. So week after week, Judy came to the meetings, but never wrote any exercise goals.

One day, she quietly spoke up, "I have an exercise bike at home in my bedroom. Maybe I could start using it a little." The class encouraged her, "Great plan, Judy. Give it a try. Just do a small amount so you don't get sick of it." Judy wrote on her goal sheet, "I will ride my exercise bike every day for *one minute.*"

The next week, Judy told the group, "I did it! Every day I rode the bike for one minute. In fact, I know I was accurate because I used my stopwatch." The following week Judy again reported success. This time, she cautiously agreed to increase her goal to two minutes a day. Once again she was successful.

As the weeks went by, Judy gradually progressed from two minutes to five, then ten, then twenty minutes a day. A year later, this person who said she hated exercise had lost forty pounds and was running four miles a day. Judy said, "I was so overwhelmed by the idea of exercising that I could never start. Making a very small goal was critical to helping me succeed."

BE PATIENT WITH RESULTS

When you faithfully stay on a diet for two weeks but lose only one pound, it's easy to lose your resolve and quit. But that's like planting flower seeds, then digging them out after two weeks because they haven't bloomed yet. Don't let slow progress keep you from staying with your plan. And if you're working on losing weight, be careful not to let your scale determine how you eat.

Anita weighed herself every morning. If the scale didn't change for several days, she would get upset and discouraged. One day she confessed, "I got so frustrated because the scale wasn't moving that I *made* it move. I went on an eating binge!" Of course, the scale moved, but not in the direction she wanted.

If staying on your diet depends on seeing results on the scale, you'll stumble every time your body retains fluids or gets stiff after exercising. Don't get discouraged if your weight doesn't show changes every week. Most of the time, a drop on the scale is just around the corner. If you get impatient, you may give up on your diet and start eating more food just as your weight was about to drop.

In the same way, be patient with changing your patterns of emotional eating. Just because you slip your hand into the cookie jar now and then doesn't mean you aren't learning anything. When you stumble with your eating goals, take out the tools you've learned and use them to sort through your emotions and take care of your needs.

When You Get "Stuck"

If you don't feel motivated, you can get "stuck" and lose faith that things will ever be different. You keep promising you'll change, but you never follow through. You set goals, but because things aren't quite in place, you never get started on them. When you're stuck, everything comes to a standstill. You may even wish for a crisis of some kind, because you're convinced that's the only thing that will get you going.

Being stuck takes on an identity of its own. Instead of working on your roadblocks, you blame others for why you don't take action. Yet if someone offers you advice, you get defensive and respond, "You don't understand my situation."

Everyone gets stuck now and then, especially when struggling with weight loss or maintaining regular exercise. But you can also get into a rut with your job, a relationship, or even keeping up your home. As you become discouraged or depressed because nothing changes, the rut just gets deeper.

Eventually you can't see any alternatives to your miserable life. You start believing you have no options and that nothing can overcome your current situation. Instead of taking risks or trying new things, you just stay the way you are.

Many people who get stuck stay that way for a long time. By holding on to their negative attitudes and beliefs, they continue to reinforce their lack of motivation. Before you can get out of the trap of being stuck, you may have to address the excuses that are keeping you there.

DENIAL

When you're in denial, you just ignore the whole picture. "My weight isn't really so bad. There are other people worse off than I

am. Besides, I'm in pretty good health for an overweight person."
As you explain why you aren't taking action, you convince yourself that being stuck isn't your fault. You conclude something else
must be the reason you can't change. So you blame work, kids, an
insensitive husband, a demanding boss, your back problem, even
the weather, for keeping you stuck.

Denial pulls the shade over your eyes and gives you an excuse
to not even try working on motivation or other changes in your
life. You become so convinced you can't change that, when someone suggests a solution, you give excuses for why it won't work.

- My situation is different . . . you just don't understand.
- I tried that and it didn't work.
- Everybody always gains the weight back, so why bother?
- Everyone in my family is this way. How can you expect me to
  be any different?
- Yes, but . . . (This is your standard response to every suggestion.)

If you've been living in denial, look closely at the truth in your
life. If you were totally honest about how you feel or what you
think about your health, would you approach your excuses differently? Think about your reasons for not making changes, then
decide whether they're valid or you've just convinced yourself you
can't do anything about your issues.

ARE YOU TOO COMFORTABLE?

Perhaps you've become "too comfortable" with things as they are
and see no reason to live differently. You like being able to eat
whatever you want, skip your exercise routine, and use food to
cope with your stress. Because you don't have to follow any rules
or standards, you can enjoy the freedom of *not* taking responsibility for your health.

You might complain about your miserable situation, but it never bothers you enough to do something about it. But are you really *comfortable*? Do you actually *like* feeling so tired or squeezing into pants that don't fit?

Maybe underneath all your excuses, you're simply afraid. What if you aren't strong enough to stay on a diet plan until you reach your goal? What if you fail again, repeating the embarrassing weight gain you've experienced in the past? Worst of all, what if you still aren't happy once you've lost the weight? Rather than deal with your fears and insecurities, it's easier to ignore them and act like you don't care.

HITTING BOTTOM

Maybe you're convinced you have to "hit bottom" before you can change. When do you suppose that will happen? And how will you know when you hit it? In truth, hitting bottom is related to how you define it. You don't have to wait for a disaster. You can create your own version of the bottom—right this very moment.

Decide you've had enough and that you don't want your situation to continue a minute longer. Then take any action, even a small one, that indicates you're doing something about it. Once you make a few changes, use them to build additional motivation and help you climb out of the hole you've defined as the "bottom."

Getting Unstuck

For over ten years, Joan had been the office manager for a large corporation. She had great income and solid job security, but the politics and stress in her department were getting to her. For months, she complained about how unhappy she was at work, yet she couldn't bring herself to change jobs. One day, as she described how trapped she felt, I gave her a piece of paper with the following words on it: *How long do I want to live like this?*

I asked her to respond to the question by the end of the next week. Her answer had to be specific, such as keeping things the same for another six months or perhaps a year. Joan took the paper home and taped it to her refrigerator. That evening, she kept reading it and thinking about different time frames.

Suddenly, it hit her! She didn't want to stay in her current situation *at all*, not even one more day. The next morning, Joan resigned from her job. She told me, "When I realized I didn't want to live that way any more, it became the catalyst to change my life. I just wish I had done it two years earlier."

Once she took the first step, Joan found other changes came more easily. Over the next six months, she started a consulting business, lost fifty pounds, and applied for the Peace Corps. She became an avid exerciser, riding her bike ten miles each way to her office and back. At age 51, two years after leaving her "awful" job, she received her first assignment with the Peace Corps and began traveling the world. Joan is absolutely *not* stuck!

SEE THE POSSIBILITIES

Being stuck is like wearing blinders when you look at the world. Because you can't *see* any options, you eventually assume there aren't any. Take a look at the illustration below.

What do you see first? Do you notice a tiny black dot or do you see a large white square?

In life, it's easy to get hung up on small obstacles and lose sight of the rest of the world. Opening yourself to new possibilities takes some effort, especially if you've spent many years looking at small black dots.

Start letting go of your limiting beliefs and look at new possibilities and explore other ways you might do things. Select an area you'd like to change and make a list of every possible action, no matter how small, that would help you make progress.

Donna's goal was to exercise consistently at least five days a week. Instead of letting her excuses keep her stuck, she made a list of possibilities that would help her be successful. Notice how she became more creative as her list grew.

1. Set alarm one hour earlier.
2. Lay out exercise clothes the night before.
3. Put water bottle in refrigerator so it's ready to grab.
4. Use self-talk from the minute I wake up.
5. Check tires on bike before going to bed.
6. Ride bike only six blocks the first time.
7. Join the health club that's nearby.
8. Hire a personal trainer.
9. Set up a reward system with a buddy.
10. Tape new music to listen to while exercising.

Let your imagination go and fill an entire page with fresh ideas. You may be amazed at all the options you can invent. When you open the door to new possibilities, you discover lots of ways to achieve your goals. Rather than getting hung up by the small black dots in your life, focus on the big white squares that represent unlimited opportunities.

How to Create Motivation

Motivation for accomplishing any goal is tied to the amount of importance you assign to it. If you consider a final exam to be important, you stay up late, turn down a party invitation, and make yourself study. When you really want something, creating motivation becomes easy. You simply have to raise the goal's level of importance by moving it higher on your priorities list.

MAKE IT MATTER

Pick a specific personal challenge for which motivation is a struggle. Besides emotional eating, you might choose something like exercising, losing weight, or quitting smoking.

Think of all the ways this problem area impacts your life. Does it affect your health or your energy? Is it harming your self-esteem? Does it make it difficult to cope with your emotions or to manage stress? On a scale of 1 to 10, rank how much this problem bothers you. Use the guidelines below to decide on the appropriate level.

> *1 = It has no impact whatsoever.*
> *5 = It bothers me some, but not enough to do anything.*
> *10 = It overwhelms me. I think about it all the time. I desperately want to change.*

Darlene had wanted to lose weight for a long time. Lately, she'd been feeling more desperate, but she was still having trouble staying on her diet plan. When she thought about how her weight was impacting her life, she came up with a long list.

- I feel miserable all the time.
- My feet and legs ache a lot.
- It's hard to exercise.
- I avoid going out in public.

- I'm self-conscious about my looks.
- I worry about my health.
- I'm embarrassed around my friends.
- I can't wear nice clothes.
- Theater seats are uncomfortable.
- My self-esteem is nonexistent.

When Darlene evaluated her situation, she said, "On a scale of one to ten, my weight impacts me at nine-point-five. Most days I feel miserable, I hate myself, and I wish life was different." As she looked closely at how being overweight was hurting her life, Darlene decided it was time to get busy. The next day, she used her newfound motivation to get started on a healthy diet and exercise program.

When you can't find enough motivation to start taking action, see if you can push the number higher on the scale. Look closely at how your life issues are affecting you, and if necessary, invent a few more concerns.

Although she kept wanting to lose twenty pounds, Karen never stayed on her diet long enough to make any progress. But aside from not fitting into her nice business suits, she couldn't think of any great reasons to change her pattern. She was successful at her job, her health wasn't an issue, and many days she completely forgot about her weight.

Because her extra weight didn't affect her life very much, Karen had a hard time staying motivated to work on it. When she looked at her situation more closely, though, she discovered a few more things that bothered her besides her closet full of unworn suits. So she added these items to her list.

- Have more self-confidence in public.
- Feel comfortable wearing a bathing suit.
- Like myself more when I look in a mirror.

- Want to be a singer in a night club.
- Want to start a running program again.
- Want to be at a healthy weight before I get pregnant.

By identifying more reasons to lose weight, Karen was able to push her level on the life impact scale from 3 to 8.

It's hard to get motivated to change something that doesn't impact your life. If you never seem to stick with your efforts, perhaps what you're aiming for isn't important to you right now. To crank up your motivation, raise the importance of the goal so it matters to you more.

PUSH YOUR MOTIVATION

Once you determine how much a goal impacts your life, think about your level of motivation for achieving it. Using the same scale from 1 to 10, select a number that represents the amount of drive you have to make changes. Use these descriptions to help you determine your motivation level:

1 = I don't really feel like working on it.

5 = I'll work on it as long as it's not too difficult or time consuming.

10 = I'll do whatever it takes to make this goal happen. I won't let anything stop me.

The higher your number, the more likely you'll be to take action. To consistently follow through with your efforts, you have to reach *at least* 7 on the motivation scale. If your motivation falls below that level, you'll probably go through many days when you won't feel like pushing yourself and you'll just let things go.

By using the two rating scales together, you can significantly increase your own motivation. First, search for ways the problem might be affecting you and deepen your desire to change it. Then consider what might push you higher in your determination to work on the goal.

Draw on self-talk, support systems, or any other means you can find to increase your resolve. Anytime your motivation starts slipping away, go back to these rating scales. Use them to invent ways to get yourself back on track and keep you moving toward success.

Light Your Own Fire

You've set goals and written action plans. Every day, you feel certain you'll get started on your diet or exercise program. But nothing happens. More days go by and you still haven't done anything. So how do you light a fire that will get you going? These next steps are almost guaranteed to jump-start your motivation and sustain it.

JUST DO *SOMETHING* . . . THEN YOU'RE STARTED!

Do you remember the first time you dove off the high board at the swimming pool? You probably stood uneasily on the board with your toes curled around the edge and waited. The swimmers behind you started yelling for you to hurry up, but for some reason, you couldn't move.

Finally, you pulled out every ounce of determination you could find and you jumped. What a feeling! After you climbed back out of the pool, you headed right back up the ladder to do it again. It seemed a lot easier that second time. But to get yourself started initially, you had to break the barrier of that first jump.

Sometimes you just have to take *one step* and mentally leap into the water. For example, if you take one walk or eat one healthy meal, you can tell yourself you're over the hump of having no motivation. Once you're started, you'll find it gets easier to continue your program and keep making progress.

Any time you lose motivation and struggle with getting back on track, tell yourself, "Just do *something*, then you're started!" Let this concept work for you again and again. Take just one step, get past the rut, and you'll find you're back on track.

THE TEN-MINUTE SOLUTION

When you can't get motivated to exercise, use this trick to help you get started. Tell yourself you only have to do an activity for *ten minutes*, then you can quit. Then push yourself out the door and take a walk, ride your bike, or use the exercise equipment at the gym. You'll be amazed at how easy it is to get yourself going.

Knowing you only have to stick with it for ten minutes gives you the push to get started. If you stop at the end of that time, you'll feel good because you did *something*. Or you may decide that, since you're already out, you might as well continue a while longer and do another half-hour. Either way, you're a success!

Never underestimate the benefits of a small amount of exercise. Even a ten-minute bike ride or a short walk can boost your energy and brighten your spirits. Even though it may not have the same benefits as a longer workout, the ten-minute solution may be the secret to getting you back to a consistent exercise plan.

SUSTAIN IT FOR THREE DAYS

Remember Newton's First Law of Motion from high school? "A body at rest tends to stay at rest, but *once it starts moving, it picks up momentum and keeps going.*" Whenever you start an exercise plan or a new diet program, you have to get past your *inertia* and then build your momentum. So do whatever it takes to get yourself started, then stick with it for at least three days, or until you're into a comfortable rhythm. If you can sustain an activity for three days in a row, you'll be back on track and able to stay consistent again.

Motivation that Lasts

Motivation isn't permanent. You don't "get it" once and then never have to worry about it again. That's why being able to build your own motivation is so important. You have to learn how to create your own wake-up call.

Don't worry about past failures. Your history with low motivation has nothing to do with your ability to be successful now. Whether you reach your goals depends entirely on the choices and actions you follow *today*.

Learn to generate excitement and satisfaction about your motivation. You don't have to wait until you have more time or more money or more energy to make your efforts pay off. Look at motivation as an opportunity, not a burden or a nuisance. You'll discover that you really do have the resources to sustain the motivation you need.

Motivation is the ticket to your journey. If you can create it and keep it going, you'll get there. Keep inventing new tricks, creating new methods, and pushing yourself, even when you don't feel like it. When you sustain motivation, all your efforts pay off—you'll see the results in your mirror as well as your lifestyle!

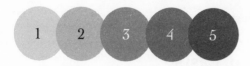

CHAPTER THIRTEEN

The Five Steps in Action

NOW THAT YOU'VE LEARNED the five basic steps to conquering emotional eating, it's time to integrate them into your daily life. Sometimes you can draw on them to handle simple day-to-day issues like refusing the tempting brownies your neighbor offers you. Other times, they will guide you through difficult life changes like moving to a new city or going through a divorce.

Using the Tools

Remember that you can use just *one* of the five steps if that's all it takes. Often, just sitting quietly and repeatedly asking "What do I need?" will help you figure out what to do next. Doing a quick review of head and heart hunger might be enough to stop you from grabbing a candy bar from the vending machine or slipping a pint of ice cream into your grocery cart.

For more complex eating struggles, walk through all five steps. For example, if you get caught in a cycle of binge eating, try identifying what you feel and addressing what you need. Search out the roadblocks that might be keeping you from taking action.

Five Steps to Conquering Emotional Eating

Step 1. What's going on?

I want to eat! (Or, I already ate.) Is it head hunger or heart hunger?
Head hunger—chewy, crunchy food.
   Pressure feelings—anger, stress, frustration.
   What do I want to chew on?
Heart hunger—unsure what I want to eat; soothing, comfort food.
   Empty feelings—sad, lonely, bored, restless.
   What's empty or missing right now?

Step 2. What do I feel?

Open my eyes to my emotions.
Do exercise "I feel...because..."
What's really bothering me? Am I sure? What else am I feeling?

Step 3. What do I need?

Where's the gap in my life?
What do I need? How could I get it? Which needs are my highest
priorities?

Step 4. What's in my way?

What are my excuses?
Am I tired, overwhelmed, stressed? Tired of working on it?
How badly do I want to reach my goal? How can I push past my
roadblocks?

Step 5. What will I do?

What's my specific intention?
What will it take? Which solution fits? Nurturing? Calming? Uplifting?
What's one goal I can do *now*?
What else do I need to do?

Instead of taking the easy way out, consider every food temptation as an opportunity to practice your skills in managing emotions and needs. Even one small success will strengthen your power over food, moving you closer toward conquering emotional eating.

You can use the five steps as tactics in whatever situation you face at the moment. Sometimes they can provide diversion or help you delay giving in to food. Other times you can use them to give you incentive or to reinforce your positive actions.

In this chapter, you'll see how real people have used these five steps in real-life situations. Each story demonstrates a slightly different approach to the steps. Feel free to adapt these ideas to fit your own needs.

A summary of the five steps is shown on page 230 to help you remember what each one includes. You might want to make several copies of it as reminders on how to use the steps effectively.

Food as Diversion

In the middle of studying for a final exam, Sara decided to buy a cup of coffee to help her stay alert for the next couple of hours. As she waited for her change, she gazed into the bakery case filled with delicious treats. Suddenly, she wanted a cookie more than anything in the world. Just one wouldn't be so bad. Maybe it would give her energy to keep studying. But since she'd already paid for her coffee, she decided to wait a few minutes and think about how those cookies connected to her current emotional needs.

Step 1. What's going on?

I want a chewy cookie or a dense chocolate brownie. Hmmm...that sounds like head hunger. What do I want to chew on right now? I know—it's the test I should be studying for.

Step 2. What do I feel?

I feel worried because this material is so hard. I feel confident because I've already covered it once. I feel happy because I'm almost done with this class.

Step 3. What do I need?

To get a solid two hours of studying done. I could get that to happen by heading back to my desk right now and getting started. I also need to get enough energy to stay focused for the next couple of hours. I could do a short walk before I go back to studying.

Step 4. What's in my way?

I don't feel like studying. (But I do things I don't feel like doing.) This class is hard. (I'm capable of doing hard things.) It's too hot to take a walk. (I'll walk in the park, where the trees will provide shade.)

Step 5. What will I do?

Get out of the bakery, go to the park, and take a walk, right NOW.

Diffusing Anger

Betty was furious! Her new boss had just tossed her monthly report into the wastebasket and told her to redo it in a way that "made sense." As she stormed back to her desk, Betty couldn't wait to reach into the stash of candy bars in her bottom desk drawer. But she stopped, realized what she was about to do, and, instead, talked herself through the five steps.

Step 1. What's going on?

Head hunger related to anger and frustration. I want to chew my boss's head off.

Step 2. What do I feel?

Angry about the way he treated me.
Furious because he threw my report in the trash.
Afraid that he won't like me or my work.

Step 3. What do I need?

To slow down.
To feel more confident in this job.
To go eat lunch!

Step 4. What's in my way?

Fatigue from not sleeping well last night.
Anxiety over the new job.
A desire to "show him" that he can't treat me this way.

Step 5. What will I do?

Go to lunch so I'm not physically hungry.
Take a walk to reduce my stress.
Write an outline of the report before I type the new one.
Remind myself that my eating won't "show him" a thing!
Once she completed the five steps, Betty concluded that eating a candy bar wouldn't change the situation and probably would make her feel worse.

Recovering After a Slip

There may be times when you slip into emotional eating without having a clue why you did it. Instead of ignoring these times, use the five steps to look back and understand how your emotional needs were silently at work, even though you weren't aware of them at the time.

Angie paused in front of the refrigerator case at the drugstore. She'd come in to buy toothpaste and a birthday card, but her eye caught the ice cream shelf full of pint-sized containers of the flavors she loved. "Oh well," she thought. "It's summer and it's certainly hot. Some ice cream would taste good." So she added a pint of ice cream to her purchases.

Later that evening, Angie settled into a chair on her patio and ate until the entire carton of ice cream was gone. When she was finished, she went to bed. She didn't even try to think about what prompted her eating. The next morning, however, remorse set in. So she decided to face what happened and process it through the five steps.

Step 1. What's going on?

The ice cream was smooth, nurturing, comforting. Sounds like heart hunger. What's empty or missing? People! I've been lonely again because I don't have many friends right now. I feel unsettled in my new job. I miss my family.

Step 2. What do I feel?

Dull—no input in my life right now.
Disappointed—couldn't get into the new apartment complex.
Lonely—missing friends and family.
Sad—weekend is over, new boyfriend didn't call me.
Irritated—my place is so messy.
Hollow—can't get energy to take care of myself.

Step 3. What do I need? How could I get it?

More people—check into women's organizations.
Connect to my soul—get back to my music, play piano.
Feel more settled—focus on living in the present.
House cleaned up—work on one room each day this week.
Better self-care—go back to my health club, take walks, eat better.

Step 4. What's in my way?

Building new friendships takes too much time and effort.
I keep living for the future instead of now.
No motivation to take care of myself.

Step 5. What will I do? What will it take? (WWT?)

Go back on my diet plan. WWT? Ask my friend to do it with me.
Find new friends. WWT? Attend Chamber of Commerce meeting this week.
Work on current friendships. WWT? Call Faye and Carla about getting together.
Start taking better care of myself. WWT? Make appointments for haircut and manicure.

Strength in the Face of Challenge

When you're dealing with major life events or hard times, emotional eating looks very attractive. It sounds like such an easy solution. At times like this, reviewing the five steps is critical to maintaining your resolve to stay away from your old patterns of eating.

A few years ago, I realized that a new employee was not doing well at my clinic. Her clients complained about her work style and her client numbers began to decline. I knew she had to leave. When I let this employee go, I reminded her that she needed to leave her files and all the educational materials, since they were reserved for use in my clinic.

About three weeks later, one of my participants brought in a stack of materials, asking how my clinic compared with one a few miles away. As I glanced through the papers, it became clear this competing program had hired my former employee. Not only that, but she had reproduced my copyrighted materials word for word on her new company's letterhead.

I was furious. Not only was this competing clinic getting the benefit of training I'd provided this employee, it was also stealing my proprietary programs and materials.

After my client left, all I could think of was that I wanted to eat. I wanted the huge "everything" cookies from the bakery across the street. Then I wanted barbecued ribs and chocolate cake. Ice cream sounded awfully good, too.

I didn't eat those things, but I sure thought about it a lot. For the next several days, I hovered on the edge of eating my way into oblivion. Finally, I decided to do the work I'd been teaching my clients for years. So I took out my notebook and used the five steps to record my thoughts and reactions.

Processing my thoughts didn't change the situation, but it gave me a fresh perspective on what had happened. First, I looked at the materials again and decided the copyright infringement was minimal and not likely to detract from my own clinic reputation. My attorney agreed and discouraged me from the hassle and cost of pursuing legal action.

Next, I pumped up my courage and called the physician in charge of the competing clinic. I was amazed to learn he didn't even know the employee had used my materials. He promised to review their brochures immediately and make sure they were changed to eliminate the wording taken from my program materials.

A couple of weeks later, he forwarded a set of revised brochures, which had no resemblance to my clinic's unique approach. Shortly after this, I learned that his new employee moved on to another job.

Step 1. What's going on?

No question here. Definitely head hunger! Anger, fury, disgust. I wanted to chew on my former employee and her irresponsible actions.

Step 2. What do I feel?

Naked—my stuff stolen.
Angry—bad employee continues to hurt me.
Afraid—I can't do anything to change the situation.
Helpless—no obvious solution.
Ripped off—my stuff stolen.
Resentful—how easy it was.
Confused—don't know what to do, if anything.
Proud—of my own materials.
Hurt, bitter—they were taken so easily.
Worried—she'll be allowed to continue.
Unsure—how much energy to put into it.
Upset—this has disrupted my life a lot.

Step 3. What do I need? How could I get it?

Comfort, encouragement—talk to my friends.
Feel safe in my work environment—move on, and be proud of my work.
Feel strong with my own clinic—beat her at her own game.

Focus for my work—don't put much energy into this issue.
Peacefulness, less stress—relax about it, be more factual, less emotional.
To not let her ruin my day—choose to be strong.

Step 4. What's in my way?

Anger—I can't get over it, not sure I even want to.
Fear—I'll lose money. Feel like I need to do something drastic.
Alone—need some support and advice on how to handle this.

Step 5. What will I do?

Talk to friends, hug my husband and dogs, pull out favorite music, listen to it a lot
Deep breathe, do yoga, let it go, walk a lot this weekend.
Visualize my strength, keep my own plans strong, continue to develop material.
Call my lawyer and business advisors; ask for help instead of doing this alone.

Sharpening Your Skills

Facing and taking care of your emotional needs rather than eating them away is not an easy task. Many times, you'll prefer to wallow in your misery or avoid looking at what you really feel and need. But to change your life, you have to do the work.

You've already done the hardest part—taking the lid off your feelings and looking at your emotional eating patterns. Now you're ready to move to another level of renewing your life.

As you dig deeper into facing your emotional challenges, you'll discover ways to hold on to your new skills and use them to conquer emotional eating forever.

You've come a long way, already. But even more success lies just around the corner. Keep doing your work and you'll find the power you've wanted for so long—the ability to successfully manage your weight long term.

PART THREE

BUILDING YOUR SKILLS

CHAPTER FOURTEEN

Life Is Not Stress

DO YOU REMEMBER WHAT LIFE was like when you *didn't* have stress? It used to be that stress showed up as an event or a problem. When you got stressed, you'd either figure out a way to cope with it or you'd wait until it let up. Eventually, the problem went away and life got back to normal.

Now, *stress is normal!* Instead of being something that comes and goes, it shifts between tolerable and unbearable. If you're like most people, stress has become so woven into your life that you routinely live with headaches and tight shoulders. You may never feel "caught up" or able to completely relax. When one source of stress goes away, you simply wait for the next one to hit.

After a while, you might not even recognize what causes your stress. Cheryl Lynn has simply adapted to her routine feelings of urgency and tension. She says, "I've lived this way for so many years that I wouldn't know how to act without it."

When people list their reasons for emotional eating, stress usually ranks at the top. You've probably used food to get through everything from divorce and family illness to struggles with jobs and parenting. Even if you've maintained your weight for a long time, a stressful event can instantly push you back into old patterns of eating for relief.

To stop this type of emotional eating, you either have to cope with stress differently or change the way you view it. In this chapter, you will explore how to view stress as a piece of your day, not a way of life. By focusing on areas where you can exert some control, you can prevent stress from contributing to your eating struggles.

The Burdened Life

Dana sank into the upholstered chair in my office and let out a huge sigh. "I am *so tired!*" she began. "No, that's not even true. I'm not just tired—I'm bone-weary exhausted." Then she described her stressful life.

Since I got promoted, my job has been a lot more difficult. I'm overwhelmed by demands. It seems everyone wants something and they all want it NOW! I probably shouldn't complain. I have a good husband and three wonderful children. But every week, I put in forty hours at work and at least another forty at home. Most evenings, I fix dinner, clean the house, and wash clothes. Then I pick up the kids from their activities, help them with homework, and see that they are bathed and put to bed.

By then, I'm shot, but usually I still have to finish a report or get ready for some budget meeting. Oh yes, my parents are retired and they depend on me for taking care of their house and their medical visits.

I'm forty-five pounds overweight, but lately I'm too stressed to even think about that. Besides, when would I ever find time to exercise? I eat too much because that's how I cope with my crazy life. I feel like I'm sinking in quicksand, but I can't figure out how to change anything. How do I get this to stop? —Dana

Does this sound familiar? When things get so far out of hand, it's hard to know where to begin. For most people, stress is cumulative.

When you keep adding more, you reach a point where you can't take it anymore. The only place you see relief is in the refrigerator.

In all likelihood, you'll never be completely free of stress. Instead of hoping to escape it, learn to separate it from the rest of your life. When you feel stressed, look specifically at what's causing your pressure. Prioritize what you need to work on, then change what you can and live with what you can't.

SET UP A "PLAY DATE"

When Chad started his first engineering job, he wasn't prepared for the intensity and high-energy pace of the corporate world. After a few months on the job, he described how much he missed the days when his life was simpler.

I can't remember what it's like to relax and have a good time. Now, my life is nothing but demands and pressure. Everything is tied to the bottom line and if my staff doesn't constantly produce, I get threatened with being moved to a lower position or even replaced. I miss having fun. I want to go back to the times when I could play and laugh and roll in the grass! —Chad

Stress can certainly take away your fun. But do you have to live that way? Maybe you just need to give yourself a chance to laugh and play the way you used to. To put fun back into your life, consider arranging a "play date" for yourself.

If you love movies but never take time to see one, designate going to a movie as a play date. Pick one night of the week—say, Tuesday—for your regular movie evening. If you need a baby-sitter, find one who is routinely available on your chosen movie night.

Select which movie you'll see, then find out where it's playing and what time it starts. When the evening arrives, don't change your mind because you're tired or stressed. Go anyway. Give yourself permission to have fun on your play date, even if you see a bad movie.

You can also apply this concept to going dancing, playing board games, listening to live bands, or any favorite activity. Set your play dates around activities that give you a break from your stress. Your real life will still be there, but now you'll have an outlet that doesn't involve using food as a way to get relief.

THINK "BROKEN LEG"

Even though I'd never wish this on you, think about what would happen if you broke your leg. Imagine all the changes you'd suddenly have to make or responsibilities you'd have to eliminate. Now pick out a few of those demands, and, using the "broken leg" approach, make changes in them right now. When you imagine yourself recovering from a broken leg, you suddenly realize you aren't as indispensable as you thought.

Don't wait for a disaster to give yourself permission to slow down. Take control now by sorting which activities are critical to pursue and which ones you can let go of.

You might even explain to your family or your boss that recent events require that you take a break from some of your demands. Ask for help in deciding which ones can wait a few weeks or could even be totally eliminated. You may be surprised at how much your stress decreases when you have a "broken leg."

Problems and Predicaments

Dr. Paul Welter, a counseling psychologist, divides stress-related issues into two major types—predicaments and problems. He defines a predicament as a stressful situation that has no easy answer or immediate solution. Predicaments won't change for a long time; in some cases, they may never change. On the other hand, a problem is a specific item you can do something about.

Having a bad job or a troubled marriage is a predicament. So are financial difficulties, being overweight, or raising teenagers. All of these situations will change some day, but for the moment, you can't do much about them.

Predicaments keep you under a cloud that never quite goes away. Day after day, you worry about your aging parents or the bills piling up. Predicaments cause tremendous stress because you can't fix them. They also contribute to emotional eating because, since they don't go away, you have to deal with them again and again.

Instead of getting overwhelmed by a predicament, break it down into smaller components or problems. In the predicament of being overweight, specific problems might include eating too many fast-food meals or not taking time to exercise. For each of these problems, you can create an action plan for managing it differently. For example, you might decide to stop going to fast-food restaurants and to join a gym so you can exercise during your lunch hour.

Janelle's father lived six hundred miles away. When he became ill with cancer, she was devastated that she couldn't see him more often. But her job and the demands of her three small children made it difficult to visit him more than once every few months. Janelle worried a lot about both of her parents and soon her stress began to affect her weight. Here's how she divided the predicament of her father's illness into separate problems.

Problem #1: Depressed about situation, eating to cope.
Action: Take more walks, use exercise to manage stress and worry.

Problem #2: Can't get home to visit very often.
Action: Call every three days, send cheerful cards once a week.

Within a short time, Janelle became successful in reducing her emotional eating. She also found that she could communicate better with her parents despite the six hundred miles between them.

Look carefully at how often you eat because of predicaments. Instead of wasting energy on situations that aren't going to change, learn to identify the problems inside a predicament, then take action in places where it will make a difference.

The "Last Straw"

Do you ever have one of those days when everything goes wrong? You get a speeding ticket, the copier needs fixing, you forget your purse, and the heel on your shoe breaks. Some days, life is just filled with hassles—the things that get on your nerves and finally cause you to lose your patience.

When you're already stressed, hassles clearly add to your frustration. Finally, one more thing happens and you exclaim, "That was the last straw!" and you head for the kitchen. Although it may seem like that "last straw" prompted your eating, you probably started to weaken a lot earlier. When events or emotional triggers are linked together one after another, your resistance drops until you finally give in and eat.

Ask " . . . and What Else?"

To identify a chain of eating triggers, start at the moment when you first ate or knew you desperately wanted to eat. Working backwards from that point, consider all of the stressful situations or people that were part of your day. Each time you identify a trigger, ask, " . . . and what else?" to help you remember other things that might have affected you.

When Jill overate on pizza one night, she assumed it was because she was tired from shopping.

On Friday night, I went to the mall with my nine-year-old daughter. After we'd shopped for a couple of hours, we sat down in the food court where I actually ate six large pieces of pizza. I think I just kept eating because I was so tired and I thought it would make me feel better.—Jill

Jill may have been right. But as she described this to me, I got the sense that fatigue wasn't the only issue. Together we reviewed the events and emotions she'd experienced earlier in the day. Each time I asked " . . . and what else?" she was able to identify another piece that contributed to her stress.

> I was awfully tired from shopping.
>
> I didn't really want to go to the mall, but my daughter begged me to go.
>
> We were supposed to go to dinner with friends, but couldn't get a baby-sitter.
>
> I was irritated because my husband was supposed to call the baby-sitter and he forgot.
>
> My husband went to dinner with our friends anyway, so I felt left out.
>
> He didn't even come home after work, but went out for drinks with them before dinner.
>
> I was missing him and I wished he had stopped at home first.
>
> I guess it's all connected to his phone call earlier in the day, saying they announced more layoffs at his company. This time, his own job is at risk.

In truth, Jill did eat because she was tired. But while fatigue was the "last straw," searching further revealed the true source of her emotional eating. Besides her anger and frustration about the dinner party, Jill felt worried about the future.

Whenever you slip into non-hungry eating, see if you can identify a chain of events or emotions before the "last straw." You may discover the situation you initially blamed for your eating struggle was not what actually pushed you over the edge.

With each link in the chain, think about where you may have slipped up and what else you could have done. For instance, did you get overly hungry? Were you trying to keep from exploding at someone? Did you skip the lunchtime walk that helps you manage your stress? For each of these issues, could you have handled the situation differently? By catching your emotional issues sooner, you'll be able to eliminate the pattern of "last straw" eating.

Dealing with Hassles

When you've had too many hassles in a row and you feel like you're ready to lose it, you need an instant way to regain your sanity. If you don't get relief, you'll soon reach a point when food looks better than any other alternative. Whether you're dealing with spilled milk or losing your job, your immediate need is to take care of yourself until you feel centered again and can resist the temptation to eat. Here are some tools for "instant" stress recovery.

Slow Down

Stress overload shows up in subtle ways. When you drive right past your highway exit, run into doorways, or threaten to kick the dog, you need to regain a sense of control. Whenever you feel pushed to the breaking point, intentionally make yourself slow down.

For a couple of hours, or even the rest of the day, consciously talk, move, drive, even clean house at a slower pace than usual. Slowing down puts you back in charge of your life and keeps you from adding more hassles on top of coping with your overwhelmed life.

FOCUS

When stress makes you feel scattered and unable to concentrate, take a few minutes to mentally shut out everything around you and give total focus to someone or something. If you're with other people, look into their eyes and listen to your conversation as if there was no one else in the world. Sit on the floor with your children and be totally present for them and their needs. If you're reading or working on a project, concentrate entirely on what's in front of you. A few minutes of total focus will calm you down and give you a sense of emotional control.

LIGHT A CANDLE

When your mind is racing and you feel like you're about to lose it, you need a way to quiet your spirit. Stop whatever you're doing and light a candle. Then sit quietly and gaze at it for several minutes. Notice the way the flame moves and shifts. Watch for the tendrils of smoke rising from it. Allow yourself to feel warm and cozy inside, as though the flame slipped inside your body and became part of your heart. When you finish, notice the sense of renewal that comes from allowing quietness and light to replace the noise in your head.

Crazymakers

So far, you've been working on ways to manage the tension already present in your life. But how often do you emotionally eat because other people make you feel stressed? Even people you're close to can get on your nerves. From time to time, they disappoint you, control you, and generally mess up your life.

In 1979, writers Bach and Dautch coined the term "crazymakers" to label people who routinely cause stress in others. They described crazymakers as "difficult people" who, in essence, cause tension and chaos in your life until they make you think you're going crazy. People who are crazymakers can show up anywhere—in your own family, at work, at social gatherings.

Crazymakers make you feel unsettled, anxious, and unimportant. These people often affect your self-esteem and make you question your own skills or competence. No matter how hard you try, you can't seem to please crazymakers or avoid getting into conflict with them.

A few years ago, I decided to play the good son role, so I called my mother to wish her a happy birthday. Her response was, "Why didn't you send me a birthday card?" So the next year I sent her a card and called her as well. She sounded upset and asked, "Why don't you ever give me a birthday present?" The following year, I was determined to do it right. I picked out a special gift, then sent it along with a card. On her birthday, I called and asked if she had received them. "Yeah," she said, "But I want to know why you don't come to visit me on my birthday." As she kept changing the rules, I got more and more frustrated. Because I couldn't seem to please her, I finally stopped making the effort. —Tom

RECOGNIZING CRAZYMAKERS

Anyone can become a crazymaker, at least temporarily. Some people slip into the crazymaker role when they're overly stressed themselves. Others seem to live that way all the time. Often you'll see crazymaker behaviors in people who have low self-esteem or poor communication skills. To compensate for their weakness, they become demanding or controlling.

Crazymakers don't play by the rules. They tend to push or manipulate until they get what they want. They may seem to be very nice, yet, at the same time, they make you feel like there's something wrong with *you*. They act like problems are your fault, but if you try to reason with them, they usually win the argument.

Here are some typical patterns that indicate a crazymaker is at work.

Surprise you with requests. Crazymakers hope you'll say "yes" before you have time to think about it. They often begin with the phrase, "By the way, can you...?" followed by a request that you work late, finish a report within an hour, or let them borrow your car. Because they don't plan ahead, they tend to catch you at awkward times, like just before lunch or when you are exhausted at the end of the work day.

Use relationships as leverage. Crazymakers use their connection with you to add power to their requests. They assume you'll give in because you want to protect the relationship. For example, your boss might say, "Remember, I'm the one who got you this job." Or your child will coerce you by saying, "Dad (or Mommy) always lets us do this."

Pressure you when you feel unsure. When they know you're hesitating about something, crazymakers push you by saying things like, "This won't hurt anything, so please do it just this one time." They may also play on your fears or make subtle threats, like "This might be your only chance" or "You do want to move up in this company, don't you?"

Isolate you from support. Crazymakers love to catch you alone, away from your support systems. Because you don't have anyone to ask for advice, they hope you'll depend on your own judgment and make a split-second decision...in their favor, of course.

Shift expectations and moods quickly. This keeps you off balance and unsure about when it's okay to say something and when it's not. Because they keep you guessing, you might think, "I'd better say yes because I don't want to make him mad."

Rob had just arrived home from a hard day at work when his twelve-year-old daughter pounced on him. "Dad, can I go to my friend Karen's house tonight for a slumber party? It's starting in an hour, so I need to know right away." *(Surprise you with requests.)*

When Rob hesitated, his daughter begged, "Please let me go. I'm old enough for you to start trusting me. Other parents trust their kids with stuff like this." *(Use relationship as leverage.)*

As he listened to her pleading, Rob couldn't help feeling uneasy. He didn't know the people she said were hosting the party, and the whole thing seemed awfully short notice. By this time, she was pushing harder: "Come on Dad, I have to let them know right away." *(Pressure to do something you feel unsure about.)*

When he asked what her mom thought, she responded, "Mom's at work, and you know we can't get a hold of her there." *(Isolate from support.)* "Please let me go! I'll clean my room and take out the trash for a whole week." When she realized this tactic wasn't getting anywhere, she switched gears. "You are so mean! You never let me do stuff." *(Change moods quickly.)*

Before making a decision, Rob decided to make a few phone calls. He soon learned the party was a graduation celebration for a high school boy. He also suspected there wouldn't be many adults present. As he kindly but firmly refused her request, his daughter realized that this time her crazymaker efforts had failed.

Being around a crazymaker can lower your self-confidence and make you uneasy. Because you don't want to disappoint other people or make them angry, you may just give in to their wishes. While this lets you off the hook, it also shows them how easy it is to manipulate you to get what they want.

You might wish crazymakers would go away, but for every one that does, another one shows up. Instead of trying to escape them, learn how to minimize the ways they influence you.

MANAGING CRAZYMAKERS

Refuse to let crazymakers run your life. Instead, learn ways to work around them and manage yourself in their presence. Here are several important concepts for keeping your cool when you run into a crazymaker.

Don't escalate. As soon as you let your emotions escalate, crazymakers know they've gotten to you. So when you deal with a crazymaker, keep your voice tone as low as possible, then speak slowly and deliberately. Avoid physical actions like rolling your eyes, grimacing, or pounding your fist.

This doesn't mean you shouldn't acknowledge your feelings. But by not letting crazymakers see all your emotions, you weaken their sense of power. Once they realize you haven't taken their bait, they stop pressuring you.

Enlist other people's help. When crazymakers push you to make a quick decision, postpone answering them until you can bring in more support. Say, "Let me get back to you" or "I need to think about this" or "I'd like to check with someone else." Because crazymakers want you to handle a problem quickly, they often withhold information. So to dilute their impact, ask lots of questions and probe for more details. At some point, they may realize you know too much and they'll give up the game.

Be understanding. When you recognize a crazymaker's style, be especially patient and understanding. Find out what else is going on by saying things like "Help me understand why you are feeling such pressure" or "You must be under a lot of stress." Partner with crazymakers rather than fight them. Even if you totally disagree, consider responding to their statements by saying, "You may be right." Then ask for more input or ideas on the subject.

Soften the blow. When crazymakers verbally attack you, go "emotionally deaf" to their negative comments. Don't take everything personally or assume they're determined to harm you. Realize their behavior is usually not about you. Most of the time, something else is going on in their lives. So instead of getting angry, mentally reframe their statements to make them sound less challenging.

If your boss snaps at you about some minor incident, tell yourself, "What that person really meant to say was . . ." then finish the sentence differently. You can actually have fun with this by "hearing" the words you would have preferred. For example, when Kimberly returned from lunch and her boss growled, "Where have you been?" she responded with a perky, "Hi! Did you miss me?"

Avoid getting hooked. Be cautious about how involved you get in a crazymaker's life. Sometimes you need to protect yourself from a stress-inducing person for a while. When you're around people who are completely stressed out, let them keep their own headaches. Listen and empathize, but don't take on their stress and make it your own.

If a crazymaker keeps making your life difficult, look at your options. Do you need to change jobs? Is it time to reconsider your marriage or a love relationship? If your struggle involves immediate family members, leaving isn't always an option. In this case, work on learning how to love crazymakers without becoming a victim of their behavior.

Anger—The Hidden Stressor

Despite your efforts to prevent crazymakers from adding to your stress, sometimes you just can't escape their assault. Once in a while, people and situations will make you furious. So what do you do when anger builds to the point of explosion?

Most people are uncomfortable with anger and avoid it as much as possible. We fear anger because it has the ability to destroy us.

And if we really let go in expressing it, we know anger can cause damage that's hard to repair.

When you are verbally assaulted or harmed by someone, you're entitled to feel angry. But what are you supposed to do with your anger? If you don't have an acceptable outlet for it, anger quickly and easily shoves you toward emotional eating.

Certainly, taking deep breaths, counting to ten, or taking a walk can take the edge off your anger and decrease its intensity. But you can also learn other ways to handle anger "on the spot" and prevent it from building and getting worse. While these next techniques won't resolve the issue that caused the anger, at least you'll be able to manage your feelings without blowing up or running for something to eat.

Take Off Your Shoe

Here's an amazingly simple way to calm an anger flare-up. If someone says or does something that infuriates you, slip off one of your shoes. As soon as you do this, your brain shifts your attention to your foot. It wonders why the foot feels cold or is able to move more freely. By the time you put your shoe back on, you'll have "bought" a few minutes of cooling-down time that will help you moderate your response to the anger.

I'm Angry and I'm also...

When you reach for food to appease anger, you might be fixing the wrong emotion. Take time to notice who you're angry at or what you're angry about. Are you fretting over predicaments and wasting energy on things you can't change? When someone cuts you off in traffic or treats you rudely in a grocery store, do you really have to carry that burden home and take it to bed with you? Of course not.

If something makes you angry, take out a piece of paper and write "I'm angry and I'm also..." then make a list of other emotions you're feeling, like disappointed, hurt, or frustrated. Identify at least ten other feelings along with the reasons for having them. By paying attention to other emotions besides anger, you'll get a more accurate picture of the situation that prompted your outburst.

The Anger Sequence

Author and trainer Jack Canfield teaches an anger-management tool called "The Total Truth Process." He has used this technique extensively in his work with high school students as well as adults who struggle with anger related to self-esteem issues.

In this approach, you complete a series of statements about your emotions based on the way the brain processes anger. With each step in the sequence, you look underneath the other emotions to discover additional feelings about the person or situation that prompted your anger. The sequence goes in this order: anger, hurt, fear, remorse, desires, and love.

You begin by describing and expressing your anger. But underneath anger, you also feel hurt and disappointment, and beneath those emotions you can identify fears. After describing your fears, you admit your contribution to the problem or any regrets you feel about it. Then you make a statement about what you really want from the other person and finish by expressing love, gratitude, forgiveness, or compassion.

When you use this sequence, you can either write your statements down or say them out loud. You don't even have to express them directly to the person who made you angry. If you wish, you can work through the sequence by writing a letter that you later destroy. What's most important is that you process your feelings honestly.

The Anger Sequence

1. Anger and resentment—I'm angry, I hate it when, I don't like, I resent.

2. Hurt, disappointment—I feel sad, disappointed, hurt.

3. Fear—I feel scared, uneasy, afraid.

4. Regret, remorse (my part in this)—I'm sorry, I contributed, forgive me.

5. Wants and desires—What I really want, desire, deserve, prefer from you.

6. Love, compassion, appreciation—I appreciate, love, thank, forgive you.

As you work through the sequence, use as many words or phrases as necessary to fully express your feelings in each category. The only rule is that you must give equal time to each section. In other words, if you write a whole paragraph on anger, you must also write a whole paragraph on each of the other feelings in the sequence. The same rule applies if you talk about the emotions. If you spend five minutes describing your anger, you have to spend an equal amount of time expressing fear, remorse, desires, and love.

Here's an example of the anger sequence in action.

When sixteen-year-old Tim missed his curfew and came home at 2 A.M., his mom was furious. At the same time, she'd been worried sick about him and wondered if he'd been hurt or in an accident. Here's how she expressed her feelings:

Anger: I'm so angry that you didn't come home at midnight. I'm fed up with you staying out late and not honoring the curfew. I hate it when you just show up two hours late and don't call to let us know what's going on.

Hurt: I'm disappointed you haven't followed the rules we agreed on. I feel sad when you disobey and it hurts me to see you completely ignore the policy we set together.

Fear: I feel scared when you don't come home because I worry about whether you're okay. I feel worried when I think about trying to set rules but not having them work. I'm afraid that you'll keep staying out late in the future as well.

Regret: I'm sorry that I yell at you when you come in late. I may have contributed to your not wanting to come home because you knew I'd yell at you. Please forgive me for not being more patient and understanding, and for not listening to your explanation.

Desire: I really want to have a good relationship with you. I also want you to honor the agreements we make. I deserve to have you call when you can't do that.

Love: I appreciate your being willing to talk about this. I love you and I understand how sometimes it's difficult to follow through with the plan when you're out with your friends. Thank you for discussing this and thinking about what else we can do together to keep our agreement working.

As he listened to his mom, all of Tim's defensiveness slipped away. He was amazed at his mom's willingness to talk through the situation rather than immediately punish him.

When you use this exercise, it's important to follow the exact sequence of emotions. This specific order helps you move through several levels rather than getting stopped by the intensity of your anger or hurt. You may find the root cause of your feelings is different from the one you blamed originally. For example, when Tim came home late, his mother felt intense anger, yet her deeper emotion was fear.

Sometimes you might realize that you yourself contributed to a situation, but you're too embarrassed to admit it. Instead, you cover it up by yelling or blaming someone else. So when you reach the section on remorse, consider how you may have added to the problem or made it more intense.

If you talk through the sequence with someone, ask the other person to let you finish your entire list of statements before responding. Otherwise, someone might react defensively to the anger phase and not let you get to the segments on forgiveness and love.

SEPARATING STRESS FROM LIFE

You've looked at the range of what contributes to stress, from hassles and "last straw" eating to tension and anger. Can you see why you might want to skip out on coping with stress? Shoving your anger away with a candy bar will always feel easier than analyzing a crazymaker's actions and deciding which tactic will help you survive.

Until you build skills for managing it differently, stress and life will continue to blend until you can't separate them from each other. To conquer stress, you also have to know what you are trying to manage. So keep narrowing it down to specific issues, then tackle the tensions one at a time. By coping with the tiny pieces along the way, you'll keep them from engulfing you and driving you toward food.

CHAPTER FIFTEEN

Healing the Tough Emotions

GRIEF, LOSS, DISAPPOINTMENT, depression—if only you didn't have to deal with these difficult feelings. Yet if you don't process and heal them, they can undermine all of your dedicated efforts to overcome emotional eating.

Throughout this book, you've been learning about "on-the-spot" eating in response to feelings that pop up during the day. When you feel stress, you eat. The same thing happens when you feel anger, frustration, or loneliness. By now, you're probably using a variety of tools to keep you from grabbing food to get relief from your emotional pain. When you recognize the signals of an uncomfortable feeling, you take a walk, listen to your favorite CD, or head for a soak in the bathtub.

But what about emotions that run deeper—the ones that don't go away with a quick doughnut or slice of pizza? Like a major physical wound, some emotional damage takes a long time to heal. If you don't address this deeper pain, it will continue to haunt you and undermine your weight-loss efforts.

In this chapter, you will explore buried wounds from hurt, disappointment, grief, and depression. When you deal with these emotions, the healing process can feel more painful than the original event. But reaching for food to escape this discomfort can only prolong your heartache and slow your progress.

Grief and disappointment don't come in neat little packages. For healing to take place, you may have to pull off an old scab and look at your wound again. But as you rebuild your life after the damage of loss and hurt, you'll discover ways to survive without using food to kill the pain.

When Life Lets You Down

You just knew this was "the one"! You anticipated a huge promotion, fell head over heels for a new lover, or got excited about a great house you found for sale. But the promotion went to another coworker, the lover left town, and the house sold to someone else in a day. With no warning, your dream came crashing down, littering your life with broken pieces of hurt and disappointment.

When things don't work out as you planned, the letdown can devastate you for weeks, even months. You spend hours contemplating what went wrong. Maybe you were certain you had met your soul mate or that the company would offer you the job. When disappointment hits, it's easy to seek solace in bowls of ice cream or a few chewy brownies.

DISAPPOINTMENT

Most people understand disappointment all too well. From your first broken toy to the partner or job that got away, you certainly recognize the ache of losing something important. Whenever there's a gap between what you wanted or hoped for and what you actually got, you have to figure out how to cope with the letdown.

Disappointments happen to us all the time. The small ones we treat as simply being an "oops" in our day. For a few minutes, you might feel discouraged because your ball team lost, the store already closed, or the sale ended yesterday. But in most cases, the sense of disappointment quickly disappears.

But coping with disappointment isn't always so simple. When a major loss shatters your life's dream, bouncing back takes much more effort. And unless you're able to take care of your needs for nurturing, food becomes an easy and appealing solution.

When a series of disappointments makes you discouraged or depressed, remind yourself to look at the bigger picture. Most disappointments represent only a tiny component of your life. For example, try to remember some of your disappointments from last year. In most cases, you recovered from them long ago and moved on to other things. Here's an exercise to help you put your disappointment in perspective.

Look for the "trade-offs." Whenever you feel disappointed because something didn't go the way you wanted, look for the trade-off you got instead. Maybe you learned or experienced something new. Perhaps a different opportunity or item showed up instead of the one you wanted so badly. Although a trade-off doesn't replace what you wanted, sometimes it presents an even better solution.

When you experience a disappointment, think about what caused it, then figure out the trade-off. Use these phrases to process a single item or event or an entire series of disappointments or losses: *I'm disappointed that . . . But here's what I got instead . . . .*

For example, if you're disappointed that you didn't get that new job you applied for, your trade-off might be having less stress and a shorter commute. When you can't get tickets to a sold-out concert, you might buy the group's CD, so you can listen to their music whenever you want.

Trade-offs don't mean you aren't disappointed. You still need to acknowledge your feelings and your sense of loss. But rather than letting a disappointment pull you into despair, search for trade-offs to give yourself a new perspective.

HURT

Like disappointment, hurt comes as a response to statements or actions that are the opposite of what you expected. When someone "hurts" you, it harms your trust as well as your sense of emotional safety. You might feel violated or disillusioned that someone would treat you "that way."

Maybe a person you thought was a good friend makes a snide comment about your weight. Or the spouse you assumed would listen to you after a hard day is out playing golf or having drinks with friends. When you've been hurt, you may shake your head in amazement or disbelief and think, "How could they do this to me?"

You hurt my feelings. When another person lets you down, you may say to them, "You hurt my feelings." But this statement really makes no sense. How do you "hurt" a feeling? Somewhat unconsciously, people develop mental rules for other people's behavior and expect them to talk or act in a certain way. In reality, when feelings get "hurt," it's usually because someone broke one of these unspoken rules.

Perhaps your mother has a rule that you're to eat Sunday dinner at her house every week. Or your friend expects you to check with her before making plans for Saturday evening. When you decide to skip the Sunday dinner or go to a movie with a different friend, you "break the rules" and cause hurt feelings.

When people chastise you for hurting their feelings, first identify the rule that was broken. Then decide whether you agree with the other person's philosophy. If your rules don't match, have a frank discussion about how each of you views the way things should be done and clarify the rules of your relationship.

In the same way, watch for situations when your own feelings get hurt. Identify your rule about the situation, then decide whether you want to hold on to it or let it go and follow the other person's rule.

Healing from hurt. Hurt and disappointment represent a loss, so in some cases, you need to allow yourself to grieve. Go ahead and cry. Express your feelings of letdown or despair. In your journal, describe your disappointments and the reasons behind them. Think about what you're missing in general and how you could get your needs met. When you're tempted to reach for food as a way to compensate for disappointment, look for healthier ways to manage your sense of loss and fill the void.

BITTERNESS AND RESENTMENT

When you ignore or push away feelings of hurt, they tend to become deeper, eventually growing into bitterness and resentment. The longer you let these feelings go, the harder it becomes to heal the wound. After a while, hurt builds into a chasm of resentment you can't let go of.

Getting hurt makes people want to hurt back. However, when you insist, "I'll never forgive that person," you sentence yourself to an emotional prison. You think you've gotten justice and punished the guilty one. But without forgiveness, there is no healing. So instead of getting even, you become the one who pays for the crime.

When Shannon's husband left her after eighteen years of marriage, she was devastated. Within a few weeks, her feelings of letdown and anger shifted into raging bitterness. To cope with her fury, she began shoving her feelings down by eating a lot more. Day after day, she consumed dozens of pastries and other comforting foods until her weight climbed to over three hundred pounds.

When she came to me for help, she immediately blamed her husband for her weight gain. "Look at what he did to me!" she sobbed. I gently responded, "No, Shannon. Look at what *you* did to you."

Because she couldn't let go of feeling abandoned and rejected, Shannon continued to suffer for years. Long after her ex-husband remarried and moved to another state, she still hadn't been able to forgive him or stop hating him. Without a way to get back at him, she turned to food as an outlet for her disappointment and hurt.

Over many months, we unraveled her deep feelings of bitterness and resentment. She slowly began to realize how her anger kept damaging her own life, but had no effect on him. Through her journal, her sessions with me, and her church women's group, Shannon was able to let go of her bitter feelings and allow herself to heal. Once she moved beyond her bitterness and resentment, she was also able to successfully lose weight.

Forgiving someone doesn't mean you shouldn't acknowledge the pain of hurt and disappointment. To recover, you have to be willing to process, feel, cry, let go, then do it all over again. When you're working to overcome a deep emotional wound, healing comes slowly and incrementally. But like the turtle creeping toward the finish line, eventually you'll look back and see the progress you've made.

GRIEF AND LOSS

Disappointment, grief, and loss are all part of life. People die, pets get old, relationships end, houses burn, and friendships fade. At some point, everyone goes through the experience of loss.

Most of the time, grief focuses on something that was taken away. But sometimes people grieve for a future they never were able to enjoy. For example, you might feel sad because you haven't found a life partner or because you can't afford to live in a nicer home. With this type of grief, you're faced with loneliness or let down as a result of what you missed out on.

Grieving positive changes. Have you ever noticed how even the improvements in your life are connected with losses? Often, things like moving to a better job, watching your kids grow up, or completing a school degree are actually bittersweet experiences. You feel like you're making progress but, at the same time, you can't understand why you feel such heartache.

Denise was thrilled her kids were finally grown and starting to leave home. When her youngest daughter left for college, she waited for the happiness to hit. But a few unexpected changes caught her by surprise.

I wasn't prepared for the silence. All the things I'd complained about— her stereo, the clutter, hours on the phone, the instant-message alert—were suddenly gone. After she left, I couldn't believe how much I missed her noise.—Denise

Sometimes you have to grieve your progress. Whenever you make a significant change, you leave behind a few people or things that mattered to you. Perhaps you miss things like the stability and friendships at your old job. When you move to a different home, you'll always long for some of the good closets or drawers you had in the old place.

As you go through life changes, be sure to acknowledge when you feel a sense of loss. Don't minimize your feelings or tell yourself you shouldn't have them. Write down the things you miss and allow yourself to grieve for what has changed. Eventually, you will move past the losses and your new situation will feel more positive.

Deeper Loss and Grief

People don't like grief. It's too deep and it hurts too much to go through the healing process. But when you experience a tragic loss such as a death or the end of a relationship, grieving becomes a critical piece of your recovery. Without doing the emotional work of grief, you risk slowing your healing or even stopping it completely.

Grief has no timeline. There are no markers such as at six months you'll feel a certain way or at one year you'll feel better. The passage through grief is as individual as a fingerprint. You will heal in your own time. But silent grief carries a high price tag. To achieve healing, you have to be willing to take grief out of your heart and place it in front of you, processing your pain through a variety of words and actions. If you refuse to let your feelings go, you can stop yourself from moving forward in your healing.

After her nine-year-old daughter was killed in a car accident, Suzanne couldn't bring herself to move anything in the child's room or give away her belongings. For nearly ten years, she kept her child's bedroom as a shrine, even down to a few cookie crumbs left on the desk. Because she couldn't deal with the items related to her grief, she had a difficult time finding healing.

Unresolved grief doesn't go away. It just festers deep inside, causing you to continue to medicate it with food or alcohol. Until you are willing to deal with your grief and recovery, you may not be able to free yourself from the grip of emotional eating.

The Journey of Grieving

Grief doesn't heal overnight. It moves slowly along a path, sometimes getting caught on the thorns along the way. If you or someone you love experiences a major loss, it helps if you understand the process of grief and how it affects people. Everyone goes through the journey in a different way. But in general, most people follow somewhat typical patterns, especially during the early stages of the grief process.

You are probably familiar with the traditional grief phases of shock, anger, depression, and eventual acceptance. While these concepts still apply, I've learned that many people go through a few additional levels of feelings. You may recognize these descriptions of grief in your own experiences or those of people you know.

THE SHOCK PHASE

With a major loss, you initially respond with intense, overwhelming emotions. Shock, disbelief, horror, and denial are all common reactions. At the same time, you may also feel numb and disconnected from everything and everyone around you. In my own experience, the final blow to losing my pregnancies came when I learned I'd never be able to have children again.

On the day my husband arrived to take me home from the hospital, he brought me a fluffy white teddy bear with a navy bow around its neck. As we drove home, he asked if I wanted to stop for breakfast at my favorite coffee shop. I simply nodded. In the quiet restaurant, I sat clutching the little white bear, never letting go even through several cups of coffee and a cheese omelet.

Five days earlier, the tubal pregnancy that had put me into emergency surgery had eliminated my chance to ever have another baby. My heart was breaking, not just for myself, but also for my husband. I wanted him to know I was all right, but no matter how I tried, I couldn't get any words to come out of my mouth.

Finally, I began talking to the little white bear. "It's okay," I said. "We're going to make it. Of course we will. We both feel sad and we don't know what to do. But we've been through hard times before, and we'll get through this one too." The bear just sat there, serenely loving back with the comfort and acceptance a teddy bear gives.

During the weeks that followed, I had many conversations with that teddy bear. Along with my loving husband and my faith in God, that little bear helped me survive feeling more raw and discouraged than I ever remembered. Little by little, I felt the pain ease in my heart and knew I was starting to heal.

When people experience a traumatic loss, they usually have no idea how to deal with their broken heart. During the first few days when a loss is the most crushing, they need anchors that help them know they can survive. For me, that teddy bear represented an anchor that helped me start picking up the pieces of my dream and move on.

During disasters such as a fire, rescue workers often use teddy bears or other toy animals to give people something to hold on to. While gripping a stuffed bear doesn't change the situation, that small anchor helps people feel more emotionally safe.

THE FOURTEEN-DAY PHASE

The initial shock phase of grief can be so painful you wonder how you'll ever survive. But if you're like most people, you experience a curious shift in the grieving process about fourteen days after the event. The ache and heaviness in your chest decreases slightly and you can breathe easier. Even though you still feel the loss, the pain lets up just a little. Whether you've lost a pet, a person, or a relationship, this two-week response appears to be universal.

At this point, you start making decisions again. You throw away the leftover food and you no longer jump every time the phone rings. Nothing's changed. The person is still gone or the relationship continues to be over. And even though you still cry every day, the intensity of your feelings gradually starts to decrease.

Along with this shift, you may also notice the return of other emotions. A new level of anger rises to the surface and "if only. . ." slips into your thoughts with alarming frequency. Often, periods of frustration and bitterness alternate with dark despair.

Eventually, time passes and you take a few steps forward. You might allow yourself thoughts and questions you couldn't bear a few weeks ago. Slowly, you begin to sort out your life and contemplate what to do next.

THE HEALING PHASE

As weeks and months go by, the crushing ache in your chest fades to a dull heaviness and signs of healing begin to emerge. For me, this meant putting away the baby clothes and blankets. A few months after my final pregnancy, I donated the baby crib to a needy family.

Yet even as you move forward with grief, you may fight an odd desire to keep it with you. When your friends push you to socialize more or to date again, you say, "No! I can't! It's too soon. I still feel so sad, so devastated." Sometimes a part of you doesn't believe you *should* heal or let go of the loss.

But at some point, weird things start to happen. You'll have days when your memory slips and you can't recall your loved one's face like you could before. You may even feel pangs of guilt because you aren't thinking about the person as often.

Perhaps you briefly forget about the empty chair and you laugh hilariously at a family gathering. Then you mentally chastise yourself for not respecting the dead person's memory. All of these changes indicate you are healing and moving on. So let them happen. Be willing to let go of your anguish and allow the healing to take place.

Getting over It

As she drove home from work, Lynn was thinking how life was good. In the past few months, she'd moved into a new townhouse, received a promotion, and started dating a wonderful man. But as she turned onto her street, the radio began playing an old Michael Bolton song that opened her memory bank.

On the night they met and fell in love, she and Gary had danced to that song. Several years into their marriage, he had pulled her from the dinner table and begged her to dance again as the song played on their stereo. She could still see his blue eyes sparkling as he swung her around the kitchen on the brown tile floor. One month later, on that same floor, she cradled his head in her arms and felt his life slip away from a massive heart attack at age forty-two.

Even though five years had passed, hearing that song instantly brought crushing pain to Lynn's chest. A tear slid down her cheek, followed by another. She pulled her car into the garage, buried her head on the steering wheel, and sobbed. She cried for those blue eyes and Gary's gentle touch, and for her sadness of having him taken away too soon.

Finally, she stopped crying and tried to pull herself together. As she snatched her briefcase and stumbled into the house, she thought, *"What's wrong with me? I should be over this by now!"*

In reality, no matter how much time passes, you'll never be "over it." Even after you've recovered and moved on, you'll always carry some leftover grief in your heart.

THE HEALING ROAD

When you grieve a loss, you gradually move down a healing road. To understand this process, imagine a long path. All along the path, at various points, are markers. Each marker represents the amount of healing you've accomplished so far.

When you first suffer your loss, you step onto the path at the zero percent mark. When you eventually reach the end of the path, the marker at the end of the path would signify that you are 100 percent finished with your grieving. If you've experienced a major loss in the past, see if you can follow your healing progress by relating it to the markers on the path.

Begin by picturing the time you experienced the loss, and then the early days of agony and emotional pain. After those initial weeks, you began moving along the path, gradually inching forward until you reached a healing level of 10 or 20 percent. As more time passed, you continued to make progress, moving slowly to the point of 30, 40, and on up to 60 or 70 percent of your healing. At the 80 percent marker, you probably feel like you've healed and that much of your grief is behind you. But this is where you stop.

I believe most people never move past that point in their healing work. That final 20 percent is where you hold your memories. It also represents the love and meaning you originally felt in the relationship or situation, even if it was years ago.

It's that last 20 percent that makes you choke up, even years later, because you saw a forgotten photo or, like Lynn, heard a favorite song on the radio. In my own life, it's what still makes me cry on Mother's Day or when I visit my father's grave site. In other words, you never "get over it" completely. That last 20 percent is to be cherished.

Knowing you don't ever have to be "done" with grief gives you a tremendous sense of freedom. Those shadows of grief are important because they remind you of the love and memories you still hold. Eventually, that 20 percent may open up less often. But when it does, don't fight your feelings. Instead of pushing to get past them and forget your loss, remind yourself they are part of your healing.

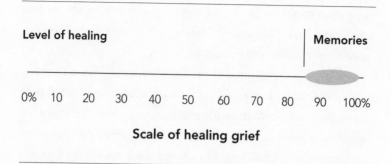

Scale of healing grief

UNRESOLVED GRIEF AND FOOD

Revisiting your memories of loss can make you aware that you didn't finish some of your work. As you went through your healing process, did you actually reach that 80 percent mark or did you slam the door on your pain? In order to keep your dark cloud buried, you have to lock those feelings behind an emotional door.

Because grief is so painful, you may have unconsciously decided to bury it too soon. If you suspect you've done this, watch for signs of unresolved grief—too much food or alcohol, a workaholic style, sexuality issues, or dulled emotions. Look carefully at the connections between your grief issues and your eating struggle. You may need to ask yourself, "When did I stop doing my work and start letting food do it for me?"

It took me a long time to face my own buried grief. It had been eight years since the final pregnancy and life had gone on. My nursing work kept me busy, my home seemed fine, and I rarely thought about babies or my losses. Because I never talked about that part of my life, most of my friends and coworkers had no idea about my history.

But once in a while, I would sense that something wasn't right. I went drinking with friends a little too often. Once in a while, depression tugged at me until I contemplated driving my car into a tree. And I ate. Whenever I felt uneasy, I reached for the comfort of food and pushed my feelings back down.

Finally, I got really tired of my food issues and frequent periods of depression. So I searched for a new therapist and started processing my secrets. With gentle guidance, my counselor urged me to pull up my old memories and tell her my stories. As I described my experiences, details began to emerge along with mental images I'd long forgotten. When I first began seeing the therapist, I hadn't cried in years. But with each memory, more tears fell. The therapist urged me to "re-grieve" those losses, crying the buckets of tears I'd swallowed along the way and feeling the pain I'd ignored. For the next few months, I spent my counseling sessions crying and remembering those dark days in my past.

As the weeks went by, I slowly healed the deep wounds I'd refused to look at before. Little by little, I began to find relief from the troubled thoughts and behaviors that were harming my life. But the biggest change came in my relationship with food. As I healed my pain, I discovered that food was slowly losing its power over me. For the first time in years, I felt at peace in my own kitchen.

I still live with my own 20 percent on the path of grief. But now I welcome and appreciate the tears because they remind me that I'm healthy. I'm not running from grief. I've learned to appreciate the love and meaning I gained from my grief experiences.

If you suspect you are harboring grief, consider working through your pain with a counselor or therapist. Even if you aren't sure whether you need professional help, have an evaluation to make sure you aren't misjudging the depth of your struggle. Perhaps you would benefit from antidepression medication in addition to verbally processing your story with someone.

You can also read books on the subject of grief or fill journal pages with your memories. As you move forward in your healing, you will replace the painful holes in your life with a powerful sense of hope.

STAYING UP WHEN YOU GO DOWN

With or without a history of intense grief, the normal disappointments and struggles of life can drain your enthusiasm and leave you feeling down or discouraged. The term "comfort food" certainly fits with the way we quickly head for the refrigerator on a down day.

Taking care of yourself on a down day is a critical piece of preventing you from using food as your therapist. So any time you experience letdowns or disappointments, instead of slipping into emotional eating, use the skills you've learned in this book for picking yourself up.

Look for the positive things around you. Find the windows in your life, throw them open, and create joy. It takes effort to do this, but if you keep the windows closed, you simply allow the darkness of anger and hopelessness to remain inside your soul.

Don't settle for just "existing" while you keep your grief buried deep inside. To get to the sunshine, you have to stop holding on to the darkness. Instead of turning to food to heal your pain, do the work necessary to find a sense of healing and peace. It's time to let the light shine again in your life.

> Grief doesn't come once
> but a thousand times
> separated by seconds
> later by decades
> but it always returns

water runs from my eyes
at unexpected moments
from a tiny rustle in the leaves
to the tidal wave that drowns me
in a deluge of tears

today it rises in my throat
but I step on it
with a glass of wine
or another brownie
and I postpone healing

it was her kindness
a free coffee refill at Café du Monde
her seeing me for real
I finally drop the shield
and invite the wind of grief

and I move in my healing
—Linda Spangle

Chapter Sixteen

Weight Loss that Lasts

IN THE WONDERFUL AMERICAN FAIRY TALE *The Wizard of Oz*, a little farm girl named Dorothy travels down a yellow brick road in search of answers to life. She really just wants a way to get back to her home in Kansas. But during her adventure, she meets several unusual characters who become part of the journey.

These delightful storybook friends were all seeking a piece of life they believed would give them true happiness. Yet as we followed them on their trip, we soon realized they already had what they were looking for. They simply weren't able to recognize and appreciate their unique gifts.

Like the characters in Dorothy's story, you may think you lack something vital to your weight-loss success. Maybe you're convinced you don't have enough self-discipline or that you can't resist certain foods. If you continue to believe you're missing important skills, you'll live in a way that makes it true.

In *The Wizard of Oz*, the scarecrow couldn't wait to be given a brain. Once the stickpins were put into his straw head, he was thrilled. It took being able to "see" his brain for him to believe he had one. Like the scarecrow, you didn't need this book to know how to solve your emotional eating problems. But perhaps now you can *see* your ability to manage this area of your life.

As you move forward in your goals, I encourage you to explore new ideas and find solutions that fit your lifestyle. But don't assume you won't be able to manage your weight until you've read the ideal book or discovered the perfect diet. Instead, reach into the "straw" inside your head, dig around a bit, and pull out the answers that have been there for quite some time.

The tin man had a different need. Because of his painful history with love and emotions, he had replaced his original heart with a container made of tin. In many ways, his armored heart is similar to the shield you may have built out of food.

Eating provides an easy way to travel the yellow brick road without having to deal with your emotions. Yet at the same time you stuff away your anger or sadness, you may yearn for the "heart" that would free you from those behaviors.

Like Dorothy oiling the tin man's joints, reading this book will have lubricated your emotional responses. Now you remember how it feels to express your emotions in ways that bring healing and relief. You've figured out how to nurture yourself and appreciate your own value. And maybe you've realized your "heart" was actually in place all along—you just needed to get in touch with it and feel its warmth.

The third character in Dorothy's traveling group, the lion, made a lot of noise but he was actually quite afraid. When he jumped toward the dog, Toto, Dorothy scolded the lion, saying, "Only a coward would bite a helpless little dog!" Convinced she was right, the lion stayed on the road to Oz because he desperately wanted to receive the gift of courage.

Throughout the story, the lion constantly protected his companions. But because he continued to believe he was a coward, he demonstrated his power to everyone but himself. Not until he drank green liquid from the wizard's special bowl could he believe that courage was "inside of him."

For you, courage is a critical tool in your efforts to overcome emotional eating. As Dorothy might say, "It's only the cowards who don't manage their weight. Successful people reach inside, draw on their courage, and use it to overcome anything that gets in their way."

So how do you find more courage? Unlike some new diet approach or exercise routine, you can't pack courage neatly into a self-help book. You have to build it yourself, drawing on your "friends"—your heart and your brain—to help you succeed.

Building Your Courage

Although you can model your courage after someone else's style, to make it strong, you have to invent your own method for getting it "inside of you." In their book, *Keeping it Off*, Robert Colvin and Susan Olson describe their interviews with people who successfully lost weight *and* kept it off. When asked about the secret to success, nearly all of the participants narrowed it down to one word: *ownership*.

After attempting dozens of diet plans and programs that never brought lasting results, most of the people they interviewed reached the same conclusion. In describing how they achieved success, they all used some variation of the phrase, *"I had to figure out what worked for me, and then I had to do it."*

That's courage! Successful people search out their own answers, refute their excuses, and figure out how to pull themselves back up when they stumble. Courage builds with action. The more times you swim across the river, the less afraid you are of drowning. As you continue to make progress, the courage inside will slowly creep outward. Eventually, it becomes the rock that holds you up and keeps you on the path to success.

CREATE YOUR OWN PATH

Think about some of the guidelines you've picked up from diet books or weight-loss programs. How many of these ideas actually worked for you? To be successful in managing your weight, you have to create your own path and make up your own rules.

You've probably heard these next recommendations from a variety of sources. Whenever you consider following weight-loss advice such as this, evaluate it carefully to make sure it's the right approach for you.

Never diet again. Over and over, you've heard that "diets don't work." Some people believe dieting causes deprivation that sets up food cravings and contributes to overeating. Actually, all the hype about diets not working has been a little misleading. In reality, diets *do* work—it's people who don't work. What got in your way was probably not the diet itself but your struggles with motivation or emotional coping.

Any effort to lose weight involves some type of eating plan or "diet." But rather than focusing on the term and proclaiming you'll "never diet again," look for a method that matches your style and your needs. Perhaps you do best with a structured plan that includes weekly meetings. Or maybe you prefer a relaxed approach, like gradually building a new exercise program. Explore the options, then find a system that works for you and take "ownership" of it.

Write down everything you eat. The instruction to write everything down has sent many people running in despair from weight-loss classes. If you hate writing, you'll either refuse to do it or you'll drop out of any program that requires it.

Recording your food intake along with your emotions about eating might give you a lot of insight. But if you aren't a "writing" kind of person, look for other ways to build awareness. For example, you might get a tape recorder and verbally describe your eating patterns and your feelings. Or you might enjoy using a computer program to monitor your progress or analyze your meal plans.

Throw away the scale. If you're like a lot of people, getting rid of the scale makes as much sense as taking the speedometer out of your car after you've had too many speeding tickets. To prevent getting caught in the future, it helps to know how fast you're going!

When it comes to the scale, decide what works for you. If using a scale makes you feel obsessed or damages your self-esteem, get rid of it or hide it in a closet. On the other hand, if weighing yourself once or twice a week helps you monitor your progress, then do it.

After Suzanne lost forty-five pounds, she continued to weigh herself every day. Instead of fretting about the scale, she saw it as an important part of her maintenance plan. If it indicated her weight was climbing, she'd tighten up on her eating plan and increase her exercise. She compared her daily weigh-in to listening to the weather report. "It doesn't tell me what kind of day to have, it just helps me know whether to take an umbrella."

OBESITY IS A CONDITION

As you already know, at the end of the yellow brick road lies a lot of hard work. There is no "permanent" weight loss. Lasting success requires constant, day-to-day effort to live within the boundaries that produce results.

In reality, obesity (or being overweight) is a "condition" just like diabetes. Once you have diabetes, you're never free of it. It can't be cured; there's no getting over it and no end to the treatment requirements. If someone becomes diabetic, they first have to work at getting the condition under control, then they have to live every day in a way that keeps it managed.

A diabetic can't go on vacation and say, "I don't want to think about my diabetes while I'm on this trip, so I'll just leave my insulin at home." Without daily monitoring, the condition of diabetes can quickly get out of hand, increasing the risk of major health problems or even death.

In the same way, you'll never reach a point where you can ignore your condition of obesity. Even once you've successfully lost weight and reached your goal, you'll always be vulnerable to gaining weight back. If you're determined to be a long-term success, you have to manage your weight condition during vacations, job changes, and other life challenges.

If you don't like thinking of your weight struggles as being permanent, you may have to work on "accepting" that you have a condition. Marian had to let go of her anger before she was able to acknowledge her risk of obesity wasn't ever going away.

I don't like to think I'm stuck with it. I've always held a belief that one of these days, I'll be done with losing weight and I won't have to worry about it anymore. Of course, whenever I've done that, I've always gained the weight back. I guess I need to get over my anger and start figuring out solutions for managing the condition long term.—Marian

Accept the solution. A decision about what to weigh is a decision about how to live. If you're serious about managing your condition, you also have to be willing to accept the solution. That means you have to live every single day in a way that matches your goals.

Think of losing weight as similar to building a savings account. Suppose you decide to save money at the rate of one dollar a day. At the end of each day, you can look at your actions and determine whether you accomplished your goal. If you still have your dollar, you can deposit it into your bank.

If you decide to buy a cup of coffee, you spend your dollar instead of saving it, so the amount in your bank remains the same as the day before. On a really difficult day, you might buy a second cup of coffee. At the end of that day, you'll have to pull a dollar back out of your bank, losing some of the progress you'd worked so hard to achieve.

Managing your weight works the same way. If you live each day in a manner that results in weight loss, you'll eventually reach your goal. On the other hand, if you overspend a little each day, your weight will eventually move in the opposite direction from what you wanted.

Follow the 90 percent rule. You can't follow a weight-management plan only half of the time and expect to see results. If you keep going off your diet because it's someone's birthday or you're feeling stressed, your weight will soon creep back up. Based on my clinic research, I believe that in order to be successful, you have to stay on your program at least 90 percent of the time or more.

That means you have to follow your eating plan at least nine days out of ten. Or if you prefer, monitor this as nine out of ten meals. Anything less won't bring the results you want. In other words, if you follow a diet plan during the week but eat whatever you want on the weekends, you probably won't achieve long-term success.

To track how closely you're following this guideline, ask yourself, "If I lived every day exactly the same way as I am today, what would happen? Would I lose weight, maintain my weight, or gain weight?" Then record your answer on a calendar or in your journal. At the end of the month, tally the numbers and see how close you have come to the 90 percent rule.

Build Your Anchors

As you work on managing your weight, develop a set of anchors you can count on forever. Start with memorizing the five steps you learned in this book. Use them regularly, either one at a time or in their sequence. Make them so much a part of your daily routine that you could follow them in your sleep.

In addition to the five steps, continue to maintain your new attitudes about food. Eat only to fuel your body or to appreciate flavors. Review the tools you've learned such as savoring, eating with awareness, and not eating food because it's "there." Integrate these concepts into your life so you don't have to pull out this book to remember how they work.

EAT LIKE A "HEALTHY PERSON"

How many times have you wished you could just eat like a "normal" person? Look around you at the people you're modeling yourself after. In most American settings, "normal" people eat too much, don't exercise, and don't care! Is that what you dream about?

Instead of waiting for the day you can eat like a "normal" person, set a goal of living like a "healthy" one. Do you know people who appear to have a healthy approach to eating, exercising, and coping with life? If so, study their patterns and draw on some of their ideas. Then write your own script for how you would do these things as a *healthy* person.

AVOID OLD HABITS

Almost without exception, people who regain weight admit they slipped back into their old habits. It starts with skipping your oatmeal one morning, then having a doughnut and coffee on the way to work. A few days later, you remember how good that doughnut

The 5-Step Plan to Overcome Emotional Eating and Lose Weight on Any Diet

Step 1. What's Going On?

Is it head hunger (chewy, crunchy food) or heart hunger (soothing, comfort food)?

Step 2. What Do I Feel?

"I feel...because...."

Step 3. What Do I Need?

What do I need? How could I get it?

Step 4. What's in My Way?

What are my excuses? How can I get past them?

Step 5. What Will I Do?

What's my specific intention? What will it take?

---

tasted, so you stop at the coffee shop again. After a few more times, you slip into your old habit of eating a couple of doughnuts every morning.

The same thing can happen if you skip a day or two on your exercise program. Soon, you go back to your old habit of sitting down after work with a bag of chips in your hand instead of walking on your treadmill.

Make a list of some of the old habits that have caused you trouble in the past. Don't forget the can of nuts or the candy bars you used to hide in your drawer at work. What about eating fried cheese sticks or barbecued chicken wings at happy hour? As you identify the habits you want to avoid, set up plans that will keep you from slipping backward into those old negative patterns.

MAKE A TWENTY-YEAR PLAN

Just like brushing your teeth or taking a shower every day, you can also define your daily approach to managing your weight. This next exercise helps you determine your exact method for sticking with your goals during the years ahead.

Think about the coming week and decide how you plan to live during that time. Will you be exercising? If so, what will you do and how much? Do you intend to follow a specific eating plan or diet program? What types of things will you do for self-care?

Now, mentally fast-forward to how you plan to live during the next year, five years, and even twenty years. Which of your current actions do you want to keep in your weight-management program forever? With those ideas in mind, get ready to make a long-term plan! See the example on page 285.

Cindy had lost seventy-five pounds and was now starting a maintenance plan. She was worried that she'd gain the weight back, as she'd done so many times in the past. Writing her twenty-year plan helped her feel more prepared and confident about how she could maintain her success. Cindy's plan is on page 286.

Never Give Up! Never, Never, Never!

You can achieve lasting weight loss! You just have to stay determined to keep working at it. When you fall, get back up. If you have a bad day and eat everything in sight, make the next day a healthier one. All across the country, people are changing their lives. So can you. Find stories and examples that inspire you, then tell yourself, "Others have done it and so can I!"

Your Twenty-Year Plan for Living Healthy

At the top of a piece of paper, write "My twenty-year plan for living healthy." Following the directions in each of the sections below, develop a blueprint for how you'll live for the next twenty years.

1. What I can do forever.

In this section, plan a variety of actions you can do the rest of your life. Don't be too restrictive such as saying you'll follow a 1,200-calorie eating plan. You aren't likely to track your calories every single day in the years ahead. Instead, plan realistic goals like eating low-fat, monitoring portion amounts, limiting alcohol, or exercising at least three times a week. Make a list of seven items you plan to do for the next twenty years.

2. Favorite foods.

Choose three of your absolutely favorite foods. Then, using the "smaller amounts, less often" approach, determine how you can enjoy these foods without compromising your goals. Decide how often you'd like to eat your favorites, then plan them into your program, not out of it.

3. Exercise.

Set exercise goals that are reasonable but strong enough to challenge yourself. Be specific about your action plans and how you'll stick with them.

4. Barriers.

Identify potential high-risk areas that might keep you from maintaining your success. Think about current issues as well as past ones that could get in your way. Add a few thoughts on how you'll cope with these problems so they don't sabotage your efforts.

5. Crisis plan.

What will you do if you begin to regain weight? Make a contingency plan for taking immediate action if you get into trouble with your goals. Determine a "red flag" weight on the scale or a favorite pair of jeans that will trigger a mental alarm and set your crisis plan into motion.

Cindy's Twenty-Year Plan for Living Healthy

1. What I can do forever.

Eat low fat foods, limit to forty grams of fat a day or less.
Listen to my body's signals for hunger and fullness.
Monitor portion sizes, keep them "reasonable."
Eat my favorite foods using the principle of "smaller amounts, less often."
Eat dessert only if it's "special" or unusual.
Push myself to eat four to five servings of fruits and vegetables a day.
Keep learning new "tricks" and approaches that work for me.

2. My three favorite foods and my plan for managing them.

Cookies, especially chocolate chip ones. Plan that I can have two cookies a week.
Lasagna. Have it once a month, listen to my body for the point of "fullness."
Cheesecake. Once every two months, have a small piece, savor it and appreciate the flavor.

3. My exercise plan and how I will make it work.

Walk four to five times a week. Do toning and strength-training exercises every other day.
Use a wall chart to both record my progress and celebrate my success.

4. Barriers and life issues, and my plan for handling them.

Stress at work. Take breaks often, keep my exercise plan strong.
Emotional eating. Review materials I've learned, add new coping skills.
Not exercising. Keep records of my progress, build in non-food rewards like music CDs or a new book.

5. Crisis plan if I start gaining weight.

Keep a food record. Count fat grams and decrease totals for the day to forty or less.
Exercise more often, up to five or six days a week.
Evaluate the emotional issues affecting my eating patterns.

Like traveling the yellow brick road to Oz, overcoming emotional eating is not an event—it's a journey. Every so often, you'll need to refuel your efforts by reviewing what you've learned, reading your journal entries, or rereading sections of this book.

Whatever you do, *never give up* on yourself or your goals. Even when it's hard, keep moving forward with your efforts to be healthy, physically, emotionally, and spiritually. Continue to move on your own yellow brick road, not because you want to reach the end of it, but because you've learned to appreciate and enjoy life along the way.

> *I'm not afraid of food—*
> *food exists*
> *my emotions exist*
> *but I've unhooked the chain.*
> *I choose to feel*
> *and I choose to eat*
> *now I'm no longer a slave*
> *to emotional eating.*
>
> —Linda Spangle

Index